THE UNTRODDEN WAYS
The story of Lucy

THE UNTRODDEN WAYS

The story of Lucy

by

HANNAH MUSSETT

LONDON
VICTOR GOLLANCZ LTD
1975

ISBN 0 575 02003 2

PRINTED IN GREAT BRITAIN
BY EBENEZER BAYLIS AND SON, LTD.
THE TRINITY PRESS, WORCESTER, AND LONDON

To Martin;   who loved us:

To Julia;   who was her father's joy and is mine:

To Lucy;   who loves all the world, and mercifully
has forgotten that all the world does
not love her. May she never be reminded.

'LUCY'

She dwelt among th' untrodden ways
Beside the springs of Dove,
A maid whom there were none to praise,
And very few to love.

WORDSWORTH

THE UNTRODDEN WAYS
The story of Lucy

Chapter 1

Soon I was pregnant again and we were happy and satisfied at my state. We hoped for a boy and planned to call him Giles. Julia was nearly two then, bright and eager and full of herself, lovely enough to make any parents want more.

Looking back it seems the grossest folly to have taken that tremendous risk a second time. One glance at the statistics should have made us hesitate. In every thousand births there would be some spastic, more physically deformed, a few blind or deaf, a number mentally handicapped—the odds were not so comfortably long as to be discounted, though native optimism would persuade us so. And we, who had never won a lottery in our lives, found ourselves numbered among that tangible minority.

But we were very happy that spring of Lucy's conception. Martin had lots of time off, and for once I was glad of his erratic times of working. I used to rail against the times when he was away evenings and nights and weekends, then without warning come home to announce that he had ten days' leave—but it did give us time when we could go out together.

We took Julia for picnics in the woods, picked primroses and cowslips in the fields around our home, and even, on sunny days, to the vast bright seashore and sand-dunes near by.

Often on Thursday mornings we would go into the tiny old market town. By present-day standards it seemed only a village, in spite of its ancient town-hall, but on market day it drew in the farmers, the small-holders, the prudent housewives, the junk-dealers and the sightseers for miles around, and the cobbled square was packed with vans and trailers.

Martin would take Julia to see the sheep and pigs, the lambs and calves, while I made straight for the junk heap—old mangles plough-shares, chamber-pots, and boxes of household odds and ends some grandmother had discarded at her spring-cleaning.

We bought fish and chips from the shop around the corner and took these to the sand-dunes. We used to keep a basket packed for just such lunches—with plates and forks and salt and cans of lager.

After lunch we walked on the shore, Julia paddling in her gum-boots, collecting shells and standing to stare at the men come on bicycles to dig for lug-worms; Martin striding ahead until he was quite lost from sight, then reappearing again bent forward in his efforts to haul some hulking great drift log he had found, or a great ball of rope, a fend-off lost from some passing ship, now heavy and sodden. These finds he thought so interesting that he exerted great physical effort and quite a little ingenuity in finding ways to get them across the sands and up to the car, and if challenged as to its possible use, would surprise one with a list of twenty alternatives. The garden became full of such flotsam, and some of it did look strangely interesting.

Martin was an unusual person. He was a marine engineer, but only because environmental accident had made him one. He had no professional ambition, and no interest in earning any more than we needed to live. For Martin life meant leisure, the freedom to pursue his many outdoor and academic and aesthetic interests. By nature he was solitary, contemplative, a thinker, a philosopher.

Martin loved the countryside deeply, as much when it was bleak and cold and wild as in its more obvious beauty. He loved walking, several miles at a stretch, and for him, a keen observer, it was always a rich experience. He preferred to walk alone, moving swiftly with his swinging gait, but since I, and then Julia, had entered his life he had adapted pace and distance to accommodate us, and took pleasure in revealing to us the joys he found in nature.

He needed books as he needed food and air and would spend hours in dingy second-hand book-shops, and if, as he went out on some errand he muttered that he 'might just call in at the library', I knew that he was gone for some hours, and was unlikely to return until they had turned him out at closing time.

Yet his real love now was home and family, and in spite of his many interests, he spent most of his free time with us, and preferred activities which we could all enjoy together.

He loved Julia deeply, and had always taken a full share in her daily care—pacing the floor with her at night, soothing her with baby-talk, encouraging her with her first solid food, supporting her first halting steps. He watched with wonder the signs of emerging and growing intelligence; he shared her delight at every new discovery; and I shared his joy in her.

The love and communion between us grew with the passing years.

As my pregnancy wore on life became decidedly more difficult. Carrying Julia I had been more healthy and energetic, more emotionally stable, than ever in my life before, but this pregnancy had quite the reverse effect. An old TB patient, never having much stamina, now I became chronically exhausted, and this, of course, had a depressing effect on me and on the family. Life was a burden and picnics not worth the bother of preparation.

Even by three months I was big and heavy and ill, and Dr Morris, my GP, insisted that in fact the baby was two months further advanced than I thought—that it would come early in November and not in January—though in this he proved to be wrong.

It was during that summer that Madame Vandeput of Belgium was on trial with other members of her family charged with the murder of her new-born baby, deformed by thalidomide. No mother pregnant at that time could have read the newspaper reports of this and other deformed babies without becoming anxious about her own. I knew that I had taken no tranquillizers, either this or any other, and there was no reason at all why I should be concerned—but there are some states of mind which are quite outside the realm of reason, and I was afraid.

So Martin and I discussed Madame Vandeput's action, as all parents must have, but we never needed to question the right or wrong of it. That it was the only right and humane thing to do was evident—she was acting on a personal moral code higher than that of the State, performing a human action more compassionate than the Christian law.

Probably it was this publicity coupled with the fact that I seemed to be making such heavy weather of my pregnancy that made us both suddenly alive to the many possible hazards of childbirth. Suddenly we no longer felt so confidently immune from tragedy as the majority do most of the time.

I have myself a sister who is congenitally and totally deaf; I have taught deaf children and children who were physically handicapped. My thoughts went back to those children, and to a conversation I had had some years before with my sisters-in-law Margaret and Catherine. They asked me about my work at the school, about the children, and about their future in society when they were no longer in a community of people afflicted like themselves, no longer surrounded by people knowing of their handicap and understanding it. We discussed what was being done, the enormous sums of money some local authorities and some charitable societies were spending, and how far this helped. I gave them my own opinion—deeply felt and long considered—that there are many gross handicaps which, though millions of pounds might be spent in elaborate equipment and many people dedicated to teaching and training, could only be alleviated in the slightest degree; and that where such gross handicap is evident at birth or in early babyhood, before the flowering of personality, the only humane course is euthanasia. My sisters-in-law hotly denied this. Life itself was to them it seemed so precious as to be beyond value—even in terms of personal suffering. But there is in life, sometimes, suffering so great as to make us forever resist the imagining, and where a babe new-born is already destined to this, there does not seem to me to be any justification for denying it the mercy of a swift and painless death. Catherine had the last word—she said it sounded all very logical but no mother of such a child would ever agree. I have since proved her wrong.

And so Martin and I discussed the possibility of such a tragedy even though there was no tangible reason for supposing our second baby would not be as healthy and bonny as our first. I made up my mind that if the babe should suffer any severe deformity I should smother it. Quickly and early and decisively. But the fear of being kept in ignorance by a well-intentioned medical staff, or of being kept under sedation so that I lost the will to take positive action, made me demand Martin's co-operation. He assured me that if our baby was not whole and complete he would tell me early.

But Julia was obviously lonely and in spite of our anxieties we were glad that she was to have a sibling. We lived in the country, half a mile from our nearest neighbour with our nearest relation three counties away. We had come here shortly before Julia was born, so we knew few local people. Julia's social environment was therefore particularly limited. I made a point of taking her out every day to places where she could at least see other people, and secretly hoped that my troubled pregnancy indicated twins—hard work at first but a quick way of getting a reasonably sized family.

In August we took a hired boat on the Broads. Julia took to the water like the true descendant of oyster-fishers and Thames bargees that she was. She wore her life-jacket every waking hour, clambering confidently about the slippery decks laughing at the motion of the boat, or she sat in the moored dinghy feeding the swans, calling and waving to every boat that passed. She ate unnaturally heartily and slept all through the night—something she had not done from birth. In fact there was little sign of the erratic, precocious, highly-strung, temperamental person that she was. Martin sailed the dinghy, fished from the deck, and in the evenings sat on the cabin-top listening to the reeds rustle and watching them sway silhouetted against the fallen sun, puffing and popping his pipe noisily and scheming to stay on another week. But I, who used to boast of the salt water in my veins, who in spite of ten years land-bound, still secretly held my sailing skill as one of the mainstays of my self-regarding instinct, I felt cramped. Five feet high I yet managed to bump my head on the deck-head, nearly as wide I got squeezed in every hatchway. There was no elbow room in the galley, no belly room in the bunk, and I felt that all my joints needed to bend both ways. The blocks cracked and the sheets flapped in the same romantic way that I remembered, the evening was as intense, but holding hands on the cabin-top in the evening I was more conscious of the rheum in my back than of the rustling reeds or the lapping water. I felt a guilty sense of relief when we returned.

Home again—to face the long long months till Lucy's birth. November passed, and our date was back to January. I felt I had been pregnant for three years. Shopping in town I saw a mother pushing her spastic child in a wheelchair, and shivered with dread. I rushed home to take my afternoon rest, and continued to go to great lengths to rest in the belief that by so doing I was ensuring a normal healthy child. In fact I probably only avoided the miscarriage which always threatened and which would have been so much better than her birth.

The brooding apprehension I had felt about my unborn child was lifted by a dream so vivid that I still remember it. I was somewhere in the East, sitting cross-legged in a circle with seven kings, all smiling and bowing at my enlarged abdomen, and I blushingly acknowledged their homage. I awoke very happy, and without analysing it too seriously I accepted the dream as a good omen—a sign that Fate would smile on the coming babe—and I was no longer afraid for it.

With December I ceased to long only for a cessation of my pregnancy and looked forward to Christmas. It would be Julia's first Christmas, at least the first that she could consciously appreciate. Two-and-a-half now she was eagerly anticipating Christmas, and every evening instead of stories she demanded, 'Tell me about Christmas'. Seeing Father Christmas and decorations in the shops excitement began to mount rapidly. We wondered how she could ever sustain her eagerness so long without reaching an explosive fever pitch. Martin sawed and sanded pieces of beech to make her a set of large blocks and I made a brightly decorated canvas bag to contain them. We shopped for a wheel-barrow and chose her first life-like doll, but for Julia it was quite obvious that the real excitement lay not in presents but in having the house decorated, in the Christmas tree with lights and glass balls, in the iced cake with candles. These she never stopped preparing for. Fascinated by Woolworth's counters she chose one small item at every visit, a chocolate Father Christmas, a coloured glass ball, a paper bell, a single string of tinsel. Shopping expeditions became the highlight of our week and Julia was happy.

During the week before Christmas Martin and I completed our shopping, picked holly and mistletoe from the copse, and congratulated ourselves on being unusually well organized. Mother arrived to spend Christmas with us and we planned a trip to the woods on the 23rd to find a tree. We knew of a worked out sand-pit on the edge of a fir plantation the slopes of which were covered by small self-sown firs. This would be our fourth Christmas visit—it was becoming a family tradition.

We awoke on this particular 23rd to find a bright sun and a sharp frost. Martin meditatively weighed the benefit of the sun for our picnic against the hindrance of the frost on his digging, and came out in favour of the sun. I was desperately trying to disbelieve the evidence that I was in labour. It was not difficult. I had had a prolonged false labour some days before and the whole course of my pregnancy had been so stormy that I found it easy to interpret this as another false alarm. Our Christmas plans were laid. Julia was so excited about it and I so anxious about parting from her, that I wanted intensely to spend Christmas at home. And so I refused to acknowledge the obvious evidence that my labour had begun, and insisted that we go for our picnic as arranged.

It was the first day of the Big Freeze—no snow but temperatures below freezing. It was a beautiful drive. The frost sparkled in the thin winter sunshine, the black earth reflecting silver and gold. The fretwork of bare branches intricate as lace must have looked much as they had at the time of my own birth, of my grandmother's, of that chain of grandmothers perpetuating back for countless generations. The inevitable pulsating of Nature ruthlessly reproducing itself gave me a restful detachment, and an awareness of the vast changelessness of the basic motivations of life was reassuring.

Choosing a tree was quite a lengthy task. We all stomped around gazing and considering their shape and size, Martin mentally calculating the strength of their roots. They grew so close together that it was difficult to find one of a good natural shape.

It was not until we were driving home in the early evening dusk that I was forced to admit the obvious. Suddenly I felt quite exhausted and I knew that the birth was imminent. Martin drove me straight to the nursing home and Lucy was born within the hour.

Chapter 2

QUITE PERFECT. A lovely replica of our first-born. The same abundance of fine hair now still in wet curls, the same fine skin, the same perfectly modelled features that Julia had been born with, and the same lusty cry. It is often said that babies come looking ugly and blotchy and crumpled at first but Julia looked perfect from the moment of her birth—and so now did Lucy. True, she wasn't a Giles, but that did not matter any more.

After that one first look there was no need to question or fret any more—that she was perfect was obvious, or so it seemed to me then, in my muzzy state. I felt happy and relaxed and looked forward to seeing Martin after the mopping up.

But it was not over yet. Suddenly I realized that I was alone. Alone with the hiss of the sterilizer and the brilliant lights. Urgent sibilant whispers came from somewhere outside. 'Blood group', 'Emergency', 'Mr Coleman at a party but coming straightaway'. And then they came in. Who were all these people? One of them started to prick my arm trying to get a blood sample. Dr Morris came hurrying over making reassuring noises. He stood at the foot end of the couch and kept saying 'Can you feel this?' I wanted to co-operate, but I did not know what it was that he wanted me to feel. And then he called to a nurse, 'Morphine'.

'Mr Coleman has a new Jaguar, he came through the Tolham Valley in 24 minutes.' It must have been some time later when I heard this—and when I opened my eyes I saw the bottle of blood suspended above me and the tube to my arm. And the room was so full of people—all handsome young men in jumpers —all Martin.

And suddenly I knew that I was dying. Knew it and accepted it. Martin and Julia would continue their lives without me, different lives, and a different Julia and Martin. I felt no emotion, only the cold realization of the fact.

'It's coming up now. 40–25. Good, good. When it's 80–60 we'll operate.' I knew the jumper boys were talking about my blood-pressure. I was interested but quite detached. Later I heard a trolley being wheeled. They talked about putting me on it, but decided against it. 'I think it's too big a risk.' One of the jumper boys came and sat beside me, gently commanding me to listen to him. He explained that they were going to move me—that they were all going to lift me—that I was to relax, not to attempt to move or help—but just to stay perfectly still. He instructed the others and about four or five of them lined up alongside me. Somehow they got their arms under me, and at the word of command all lifted and moved me together. They must have moved with military precision—guardsmen could have been proud. I was not conscious of moving at all, only of being moved. I breathed deeply and was away.

Martin, Martin, why wasn't he here? I was petulant and indignant and very uncomfortable. I retched. My throat hurt and my mouth was dry and sore. The nurse sitting beside the bed watching the blood-drip attended me. But when I asked for a drink she only told me to go back to sleep. 'Where's Martin I want to see him,' I demanded. But she only urged me to sleep again. I realized then that Martin was not there, had not been there with the jumper boys. They were all doctors and had worked for several hours to keep me alive—but Martin had not been there. I wept with self-pity and indignation. I retched again and demanded that they phone for him immediately. They refused. 'You are separating us,' I accused them. 'It is our joint life together which is threatened, but you separate us when you force us to experience the dangers separately.' They gave me another injection and I tossed and dozed and called for Martin intermittently till morning. And then Dr Morris was back again after only a few hours' sleep. He assured me that all was well now and stopped the drip. Certainly, he said, I could have a drink and see Martin—and when I asked about the baby he said he hadn't seen her again yet, he had only come in to see me. An evasive answer but it did not worry me then.

I phoned Martin and heard his dear familiar voice quoting our number, and Julia chattering in the background. I imagined him busy with her dressing and breakfast. 'Where the hell are you?' I demanded, my voice trembling with the anger and hurt of his not being there, and his soft gentle voice explained that he had phoned an hour before and had been told that I was sleeping peacefully, and he was not to come for an hour or so. He would be coming as soon as he had settled Julia to her breakfast. I was too ashamed to speak.

I turned my head away from the door as he came in—too proud to let him see my tears, too angry and too ashamed, and desperately needing him. He came right round the bed and sat down and took my hands and dropped his head down on me hiding his face. And my fingers caressed his thick curly hair and I raised his head and we kissed; and it was all right again. I went on vomiting the foul brown ether vomit—but it didn't matter, Martin was with me again.

It was not until the evening of that day, when Lucy was nearly a day old that I asked to see her again. I was shocked at the apparent change in her looks—now she was purple-coloured with an oddly shaped face. Her forehead was very narrow, almost pointed, and her jawline almost the width of her shoulders. Small film-covered eyes, rather Chinese-looking, barrel-chested, and with one crumpled ear. I insisted on completely undressing her to make sure she was whole, and satisfied myself that her very odd looks were entirely due to her too-quick delivery. I loved her instantly, which I knew was not a thing to be taken for granted.

When Julia was born I had no automatic feelings of maternal love for her, yet she was a baby we both wanted. During that pregnancy—such a happy time—I had attended relaxation classes and studied the Grantly Dick Read method of natural childbirth, and I approached that new experience confidently. The shock of those long hard hours of pain was perhaps the greater for that. As labour dragged on and on endlessly the new loved life within me came to be regarded instead as an alien cancerous obstruction which would not leave me till it had sapped my own life energy quite away. And so when that alien lump was finally ejected perhaps it was not surprising that I felt no love for it. But I loved Lucy instantly.

On Christmas morning Martin brought Julia in to see me. She chatted excitedly about her stocking and presents and the tree with lights; obviously her thoughts were full of Christmas and I was glad then that the festivities dulled her awareness of my absence. She came in to see me every morning, and when Christmas was waning there was the excitement of all that snow. Soon there was a foot of snow everywhere and Martin got out the toboggan and hauled her nearly a mile down the hill to visit me. Indulgently he hauled her back up again as well, and Julia was delighted.

Dr Morris continued to come in to see me every day and I was mildly astonished at his persistence. After the infusion of all that blood I felt fine and made a much more immediate recovery than I had with Julia. And so, when, a week after the birth, I heard him phone to say that he was coming again, and considering that it was Sunday, and snowing, and the roads ice-packed, I vaguely began to wonder if after all there was something I did not know about. Even then I wasn't worried about the baby. Every day I nursed her in my arms to feed her and she sucked lustily enough and then fell asleep—as perfect babies should and Julia never had. I boasted to the nurses about the great improvement this baby was on my first—who had lain awake and crying for 19 hours out of every 24, and never had taken more than a fraction of the food prescribed for her. As that week went by Lucy's looks had improved tremendously. The purple faded, the crumpled ear straightened and the face generally took on a more usual shape. She looked now quite pretty to me—and I did not doubt that she would look at least quite ordinary to anyone else. Every evening, when Martin came alone, we had her cot in from the nursery and Martin took her in his arms and paced up and down the tiny room with her, talking baby-talk. She opened her little round eyes wide and looked about alertly, appearing to respond to him, and we said she was going to be as bright as Julia.

And so I felt a little uneasy when I heard Dr Morris was coming again that Sunday just a week after Lucy's birth. He came in wearing heavy gum-boots and a duffle-coat. His dress was reassuring; so were his words. 'Yes you've made a wonderful recovery—yes you can go home soon. No, we are not at all worried about you.' I wondered why he didn't go. 'But we are just a little concerned about the baby.' I waited to hear more, not really worried. 'We think she is a little mongol.'

Of course I didn't believe it. He was talking nonsense. I cross-examined him—asked on what evidence he based his assumption. He said 'Her looks'; which seemed most inadequate to me—evidence I could readily discount. I pointed out to him the great improvement in her looks during the past week—the extreme normality of her as a baby. But he gently insisted.

When he had gone I told myself what a fool the man was. I comforted myself by recalling all the separate instances in which I had known a doctor to be wrong—and in my long medical history there had been a few. I rejected the idea completely and felt indignant that he should trouble me with such silly notions. But I had to tell Martin. I must not worry him—because it was not true—but I had to talk with him about it. I phoned. He was out in the snow with Julia building a snow-man and Mother called him. I assured him that everything was quite all right, but if he possibly could get away would he come now? Sensing or guessing that something was wrong he simply said, very firmly and gently, that he'd come right away.

He was there within minutes. Deliberately I kissed him slowly and waited some seconds, mustering my own control. Calmly I told him that the doctor had been and what he had said. In the same breath I told him what nonsense I thought it—and brought out all my evidence, both of Lucy's normality and of doctors' fallibility. Silently he heard me out and we held each other close. Then he buried his head in my shoulder and said, 'She's a lovely baby, darling, she's a lovely baby.' But he said it quietly and urgently—assuring me that we need not feel other than proud of her. No passionate denials of the diagnosis, no indignation, only acceptance. And a cold fear took hold of me. 'But you can't think—you don't mean—it couldn't possibly be true?' And holding me very tight he answered slowly 'I think—perhaps—it might.' And then I knew that it was.

The long long afternoon. Soon I must wash my hair—but not too soon—for what should I do after that? Desperately I stuck to my determination to behave normally, to do exactly as I would have done; only now I could not think, could not imagine how my time and thoughts would have been occupied if not by this. This imagining, this restraining of the urgent compulsion to act. I wanted to pick her up in my arms and hold her and squeeze her till that tiny frail heart ceased to beat. Oh let me do it now—now—I can't wait Martin—let me do it now. But no, no, Martin said no, not yet; I have got to think of the consequences, got to think what they will do to me if I don't plan it carefully, do it secretly. I must wait till tonight. Now I must wash my hair. Wash it and set it with pins and dry it with the hair-dryer, then Martin will be here. Martin will come and we shall have Lucy in. We shall have her to love and to cuddle the whole evening, an evening to give her a life-time's loving. Oh Lucy, my darling, let me love you now, in secret, even from Martin. I'll get her now—open the door softly, softly, and go to the nursery. My God, it's locked. My own baby and I can't get to her. My God, they've locked my own baby away from me. Go back, go back before they see you. Why am I on the floor, why won't my knees stiffen so that I can stand on them? My legs are like a marionette's, all limp and crumpling beneath me. Now I'm better, now I'll be calm, control myself. Now I'll wash my hair and set it just so as if—as if——

And I washed my hair and dried it though I could not really

bring myself to set it very carefully and at last evening came and Martin arrived.

I can't remember now how it was. He came and we talked— but what did we say? I told him what I had to do, what I so urgently and instinctively and desperately felt I had to do. And Martin agreed with me that it was best. It came to us both as instinctively as to a jungle cat, that the runt must not live. It must be killed quickly and decisively; both for its own sake and for ours. But not just now, Martin said, not tonight. Wait, wait until we get her home, then she will be our own. Martin argued frantically to quell my feelings of urgency. In our complicated society we were not free as the jungle cats to act on our own instincts or convictions, however compelling they were. There was another law against this action we knew to be so right, and the consequences for breaking it would be harsh. What price would I pay? What price Martin? And what the penalty for my little Julia? To be deprived of her mother for many years, perhaps all her childhood years—was it possible? I must be careful. I must restrain myself. I must do what my own con-science told me was right, but I must be sly and cunning as a fox. Right as I knew myself to be, I must act as stealthily as any criminal to avoid discovery. Already I felt an alien from society, an outcast. Already I was changed—separated from all humanity —alien mother of an alien child. Outcast.

Chapter 3

THE COLD AND the snow deepened. Sister warned me that we should have to be very careful to keep Lucy warm on the journey and at home. She would need a constant temperature of 70 degrees and must not be allowed to get cold. She warned me that Lucy was a difficult feeder and said what a problem it was to get baby mongols to suck. She brought Lucy in and we dressed her in layers and layers of woollen garments and sister put a hot water bottle in the carry-cot she was to travel in. A nurse brought in the paraphernalia of bottles and teats and drops for her eyes and her weight-card. She had been seven-and-a-half pounds at birth, and now, at ten days old, weighed only six-and-a-quarter. Sister assured me that this was quite usual. 'Mongols,' she said, 'are always slower to regain their birthweight than ordinary babies. Don't worry, she will regain it in time so long as you make her suck.' How could she—how could she go to such lengths to assure me that Lucy would live? Didn't she know how my heart lifted when I knew of the drop in Lucy's weight, rejoiced at how frail she was, of how even the cold on the journey home was a hazard? Sister went on and on giving little tit-bits of advice on caring for her. What could I say to her? 'I don't want to know, I don't need to know—Lucy will die, die, die. I shall never need your advice.' Two of the nuns came in to say goodbye. They brought a box of babies' hand-made dresses left over from their autumn sale. 'Wouldn't you like to buy one for the baby?' I handled the lovely little garments regretfully, Lucy would never need them. But I must not let them know, must not let them suspect my intentions. I had better buy one. I chose the very plainest with trembling fingers and wished they would go. 'And you must bring her back to see us,' they were saying, 'in the summer. We shall always be pleased to see one of our babies,

EVEN if she is a mongol.' I shall never forgive her for that 'even' I thought bitterly.

At last we were actually saying goodbye. How hard it was to eject those few conventional words of thanks. But harder still to listen to their murmured words of sympathy. Superficial sympathy, expressed in platitudes.

We drove slowly out of the gates, the tyres crunching on the packed ice—and I felt a great surge of relief. I urged Martin to stop somewhere on the short journey home so that we could talk. He seemed impatient to get back, but I knew that once there, with Julia's constant chatter and the presence of my own mother, there would be no privacy for long unendurable hours.

'Now,' I said when he stopped and turned to me. 'Now I will do it. Let me do it now.' Perhaps, if Lucy had been in my arms instead of in her carry-cot, I would have squeezed her firmly and pressed her closely to me till she lay inert. As it was I needed Martin's co-operation, and perhaps the reaffirmation of his moral support. Again he restrained me. He started to talk—about it and about. I felt as if I were growing physically smaller and smaller as he spoke. 'You remember, you remember what Dr Morris said . . .' He spoke urgently, gripping both my hands, his face lined and taut. 'That, that . . .' he hesitated, unable to bring himself to say the word, 'they . . . are highly susceptible to infection. You know what will happen. Julia will go to nursery school and catch every childish infection that is going—you know she will; all the children there are constantly getting colds and tummy upsets, and Julia is bound to get mumps or measles or whooping cough, she's bound to pick up something before the summer, and with Lucy so small and so susceptible she won't have any resistance—it will develop into pneumonia and she will die. Leave it, leave it my dearest. We'll just love her for the little time that we have her—she surely won't live for more than a few months.' I sat shrivelled up, feeling small and old, cold and numb, cast out, not just by society at large, but by Martin too —even he. I knew that I was on my own. Martin was taking the easy way out, just hoping that things would go the way he wanted—but my experience of life had taught me not to put my trust in a benign Fate. I was desolate.

We drove on, and as we stopped in front of the window I was shocked by the brightness within, the lit Christmas tree and the bright colours in the room. I had quite forgotten about Christmas. Julia greeted us excitedly and with a heart of ice I handed the baby to my mother. We had not told her about Lucy, and I could not bear her to know. In the past I had brought enough sadness and suffering to my mother and I could not add to it now. Years ago, when I was only a few weeks out of training college I had gone down with advanced tuberculosis. My father had died only months before and Mother and my young brother and sister had looked to me to support the family. It was more than three years before I got back to teaching, and then only another two before I broke down and was back in sanatoria again. And in all that time my mother had suffered for me, visited and cosseted me, so I could not bear to bring this other hurt to her now. And so I handed Lucy to my mother, my heart a sliver of ice, and waited. Mother looked keenly into her face and examined her fingers and feet. She snuggled her tightly and felt the shape of her tiny round head. And then she laid her down in her cot and said 'What a lovely baby she is. She looks just as Julia did.'

Julia could not wait to show me the tree, squealing excitedly and pointing out every separate bauble. Kneeling beside her and the tree I almost could not bear the contrast between her warmth and lightness of spirit and my own frozen soul. I closed my eyes and put my arms around her but she thrust me away carelessly, dashing to get her new wheelbarrow to show me. It was full of dolls and teddies and vegetables—'their dinner Mummy'—and clattered as she trundled it about. The noise echoed in my head and my thoughts raced with it. I was alone in my resolve, but it was as strong now as ever. Julia will continue to grow up light-hearted, prattling all the way, and Martin will go about his work relaxed and confident. We will be a united family again as before, our lives will continue as if she had never been. Tonight, this very night, I shall kill Lucy.

One o'clock. The church clock struck again. One o'clock already, surely not a whole hour since it struck twelve. Martin breathed steadily, his body hunched and turned away from me. He felt hard and strong but I knew that he was not so strong as I. I was made of steel. But the night hours were passing. Two o'clock struck, already, and I haven't thought it out yet, haven't sorted it out, haven't considered it carefully. Now I can think about it, now, now, after all those hours of chatter from Julia, the polite remarks to Mother discussing weekend meals and shopping bills —oh God, how did I endure it when all I wanted to do was think; think about Lucy? But now I can think—now. What shall I think? How to do it—how? I could just bring her into bed with me and squeeze her firmly—but Martin might wake. Martin must not know, not now—I must do it alone and not even tell him, and if anything is discovered he will not be involved. He cannot face it now, this thing which he knows is right—he cannot face the doing of it. It is hard to do something that you know all society will condemn you for. So he hopes, hopes for his baby's death—but cannot bring it about. And so I must do it alone. Alone and now.

I crept out of bed and lifted Lucy from her cot. She was so warm and soft, breathing so gently and peacefully. I cuddled her greedily—I had not known how hungry my arms were for her— and took her downstairs. I switched on the electric fire and sat rocking her, rocking and crooning, not to comfort her, but myself. I wanted to love her a little before she went—wanted to have her to cuddle and to love. How do you get a life-time's loving into a single night?

Five o'clock! It's almost time—time my Lucy was gone. But how? I had not been thinking—all this time that I've spent cuddling Lucy, I've not been thinking it out. I walked to the window and lifted the curtain, the chill striking us through the glass. The snow was still falling and a bitter east wind blowing. This was how—this was the way, the obvious only way. This is why it has been snowing all the time. The snow had come for Lucy.

I laid her down in her carry-cot and took off the little protective hood and coverlet. I lugged the heavy and cumbersome thing to the kitchen door and awkwardly lifted it outside. I was trembling so much that I could not put it down steadily and I was surprised that the bump did not wake her. I came back into the kitchen and stood with my face pressed against the window watching her. She stirred a little, but did not wake or cry. My teeth were chattering so violently and uncontrollably that I stuffed the tea-towel in my mouth to stop the noise. Then I could hears sounds coming from the room above, unmistakable sounds of Mother getting up as she often did in the early hours. Quite without thought I dashed outside and brought in the carry-cot. I lifted Lucy out and took her in beside the fire to warm her. And I knew then that I could not do it while my own mother was there in the house.

And so her life continued for a spell. My determination never wavered in those early days, but my mind seethed always with plans for how and when. My thoughts and emotions were in turmoil—but desperately I tried to act out my usual rôle. I did the washing and ordered the groceries and cooked the meals and tended Lucy; and even, hardest task of all, played with Julia when I could no longer refuse her. The days were full with domestic activity and frantic superficial chatter—when underneath I burned and yearned for the night, the long quiet hours of the night when I could think and plan and think and plan again, and creep downstairs with Lucy limp in my arms to give her her brief loving, and to plot and scheme again. Martin slept so heavily he never knew of the hours I spent awake. It seemed as if I hardly slept at all. It never occurred to me to take one of the sleeping pills Dr Morris had left. I never wanted them—those thinking loving hours were too precious.

But my act did not deceive my own mother. I began to catch her fixing me with a long intense stare and I knew that she guessed something of what I was feeling. I had to tell her. But how could I hurt her so? There came a time when quite without warning I burst into tears on her shoulder, and I spoke to her about Lucy. But I did not tell her simply that Lucy was a mongol. I told her what I determined should be true and what I thought would be acceptable to her—that Lucy was soon to die. I told her that the baby had a defective heart and that the doctors had told me she could not survive more than a few months. In fact, mongols often do have a heart defect, though I did not know about Lucy's. Mother took this as I knew she would, with stoical acceptance. She pointed out to me what a blessing it was that Lucy's deformity was one of which she would die early. How much worse to have had a child suffering from some gross physical or sensory handicap to be carried for a full life-span! Death was no pain to Mother, death was the release from suffering and that was blessing enough.

We talked and talked. She had noticed the several little oddities about Lucy that only a mother—or a grandmother— would notice, and now she spoke of them. I went on to tell that Lucy was a mongol, but I made it sound quite secondary to her heart-condition, and, confident that Lucy would not live long, Mother was untroubled. Indeed, she had only the vaguest notion of what a mongol was. She comforted me. She told me I had nothing to weep for. I had been given a sweet little baby to love and to cherish for all its short life. No harm, she said, or suffering was laid up in store for Lucy when I was not by. Although all her philosophy was based on a false premise, yet I was comforted. How satisfying it was when Mother picked Lucy up and pointed out all the obvious signs that Lucy was not normal. How very floppy her head was, how very small and frail she looked, how blue and mauve her hands and feet, how noisy and irregular her breathing, how sleepy always—never waking voluntarily for food, never crying at all, and how often that blue shadow came around her lips and nose. "Oh yes, it's obvious," said Mother, "that she is too frail to survive long."

What hope soared in me! Suppose after all Mother was right? Suppose Lucy really did have a malformed heart? After all, many mongols did. Why had I not thought of it before? Perhaps after all I would not have to kill her, because she will die naturally, just as Martin said. But how could I be sure? I had to have more information. Somehow I had to find out a lot more about the condition called mongolism. I was in a fever and trembling again—but this time with excitement and hope.

Chapter 4

AFTER A FORTNIGHT or so Mother went home and Martin and I both felt relieved at being alone together. At last we could talk freely and intimately of our feelings about Lucy. I turned to him now for solace, and he to me.

Martin was as anxious as I, but I think he was better able to contain his anxiety; he was not so desperate as I to have the situation instantly resolved. But now we could talk. I told him of my new hope, that perhaps after all Lucy was too frail to survive—but surprisingly he was not so optimistic as I. We went over and over all the little details of her behaviour and condition, but Martin did not think it was anything she was likely to die of. We dared to speak again to each other of our earlier intentions. We went over and over all the possibilities, trying to imagine our lives as they would be if Lucy lived. We imagined the subtle rejection a school-girl Julia would experience because of her sister; the continual and perpetual limitation of our lives because of her, and the slights and frustration and loneliness she must herself endure. All the world loves a baby—even a mongol baby—but who will love or even accept an ungainly growing idiot? Many—even most—will shun her, and many will shun Julia because of her. Would a teenage Julia be happy to bring her friends home? And what would they think of Lucy or—more important—what would their parents think of her? What would be the quality of Lucy's life if she lived? And what the quality of Julia's, of Martin's, of mine? Was the price in our lives worth the gain in hers? Or was the future for her so uncertain as to make it better to ensure her peace now? For Lucy the greatest handicap of all is simply that she is socially unacceptable. The fault lies not in Lucy but in society. But there is nothing I can do about society—I can only protect Lucy from it.

We hardly mentioned the possibility of sending her away to an institution—the thought was utterly repugnant. Her death we could face, and we could talk about her life with us, and the cost; but that only other possibility we could not even consider —we could not do that to our dear little Lucy.

Our fears possessed us utterly. We thought and talked till we succumbed to the heavy dreamless sleep of the exhausted, and then we thought and talked again as soon as sleep and work and household chores regenerated us. We worried about the adult Lucy. Who would look after her when we were no longer able? Like most parents of mongols we were already nearing our forties—was Julia to take over where we left off, just at the time when she should be starting a career or a family of her own?

We fretted about the effect of Lucy's existence on Julia. After all I had had first-hand experience of being the older sister of a handicapped child. Melanie, my little deaf sister, or deaf and dumb as it was called then, had lived at home with us, deeply loved by my parents and by me and our whole family life centred around her. We moved away from the village where we lived and went to the outskirts of a dirty bustling city so that Melanie could attend a special day school. I left my little village school —two class-rooms separated by a curtain—and went to an enormous four-storey barracks which seemed to hold all the children in the world. Children of a foreign world, in which I was the stranger and strange.

There were lots of children living in our road who used to play in groups in each other's gardens or in the street, but Melanie could never join in their activities, so I excluded myself too, to stay with her. Mother was constantly anxious about Melanie—for her physical health and safety, for her happiness at school and at home—and it was too easy to allow a loving and willing older sister to accept the rôle of playmate, inter-preter, teacher, guardian and comforter. As time went by I slipped more and more exclusively into that rôle, and had no other friends. I took Melanie to the school-bus before going to school myself, came home alone and then played with and amused Melanie almost all the out-of-school hours. As soon as

2

the long summer holiday came we, Melanie and I, went to stay with our grandparents in the village we had left. There at least I had cousins to play with, and Grandmother was much more relaxed about Melanie than Mother was. Looking back it seems that those summer holidays with Grandma were the only care-free periods of my childhood, the rest is strained and tense. No, I did not want Julia's life to be as warped as mine had been. If Lucy lived we would have two handicapped children—one by nature, the other by that circumstance.

Euthanasia, we knew, was for us the right and best course to take. But euthanasia is a suspect word, a word that makes people uneasy, a word which quite overwhelms people. Curious that people are not so overwhelmed at the responsibility of bringing a child into the world as at taking one out; an attitude which seems reasonable when conception and birth and survival are considered acts of God, but hardly tenable in our present know-ledge of contraception, family-planning and world over-popu-lation, when conception is as purposeful as avoidance.

If Lucy should die a natural death, all the world would say 'It was for the best'. Why is it that what is right if it happens by accident cannot be right if brought about by design? Euthanasia, a word not even recognized in law. In law what we wanted to do, and felt morally justified in doing, would be murder, and the penalties were harsh; so harsh that we would all suffer as much by breaking the law as by conforming to it. Is there no country in the whole world so enlightened as to permit euthanasia for children such as Lucy?

Is it such an alien idea? I have lived through a world war—a contract between national governments to slaughter each other's subjects—the basic aim to see who can annihilate most. In war a man may kill—a child's father, a mother's son, students, workers, doctors, thinkers, all disguised in a common uniform; or by bombing may kill those very children; but in the name of war this is right, this is just, this is even so commendable as to earn him a medal; but in peace, in the name of compassion and mercy, let that same medal-winner kill his own deformed new-born babe, and it is murder and society condemns him.

But there were practical things to be done and my heart sank as Martin spoke of them. We had made no decisions, reached no conclusions, and for the moment Lucy lived. We could not, Martin said, keep the truth from our friends and relations much longer—soon we must tell them; and soon too I must take her along to the baby-clinic as Dr Morris had told me to do.

The cold intensified and the snow piled up. Day after day it was the main news headlines and reporters vied with each other in thinking up titles for the Big Freeze. Living as we did on a steep exposed hill well out of the town, it was often quite impossible to get out. Snow-ploughs became the most frequent traffic on the road, and often they were hardly visible in the dark swirling snow, and behind the ever-growing banks of packed snow that made the road daily more tunnel-like. We had every excuse for not taking out a new-born babe, and our few friends every reason for not visiting. But there were one or two determined characters who called in, and I went through an agony of superficial chatter, delaying the dreaded moment when I would have to take them up to see Lucy. I could not bring myself to tell them, so I contrived to keep Lucy well-covered in her cot, whisking visitors in and out quickly with instructions not to disturb her, so that they could have got no more than a vague impression of a baby's shape under the coverlet.

I put off telling the truth to anyone. For one reason I shirked the pain of telling them, and for another, I still suffered the occasional overwhelming hope and doubt that it was after all a wrong diagnosis. The wild hope would surge up and leave me trembling with excitement and I would rush to pick up Lucy and examine her closely all over again. Only too often now I saw her little half-webbed toes, and the short little fingers and the flat little face, her head lolling limply and her emaciated body. I had to acknowledge that obviously something was wrong with her, but surely it might be something different, some obscure condition that, once diagnosed, could be treated. But I knew this to be only a straw I was clutching.

There was that first occasion when Miss Fraser called. Miss Fraser was our health visitor and I knew and respected her from the many visits she had made when Julia was small. As soon as I saw her half-smiling on the doorstep hope surged within me again. Here was someone who really was an expert at new-born babies. Why, she had probably handled and observed a hundred times as many as my GP. I knew her to be competent and wise and unprejudiced, and I saw my opportunity to get another opinion about Lucy. Immediately, I asked her what she knew about Lucy, what doctors' reports she had had, and she told me that she knew nothing but that I had given birth to a baby girl on such a date. I told her that I wanted her to examine Lucy carefully and tell me what she thought about her. She lifted Lucy gently on to her lap. She examined her slowly and carefully, saying nothing. I could not bear her silence any longer—why didn't she say something? 'What do you think? What do you think?' I demanded urgently, but she was quiet and evasive, and I had to tell her then what the doctor had told me. And she spoke quietly and gently to me, almost as Martin had done: 'I think, perhaps, he is right'. And I felt my heart become a cold hard lump, like the lumps of packed ice thrown out by the snow-plough.

That night I crept downstairs again with Lucy in my arms. I had to act. I thought she would die if I made her cold, but I could not bear to hurt her. So I filled the sink with tepid water and plunged her in, clothes and all. My own water splashed my legs as I held her, and Lucy gave a deep gasp. I held her head above the water, wanting to hold it down but unable to. I lifted her out and placed her, with her sopping dripping clothes into the cold pantry, and left her. But Lucy cried. A pathetic feeble cry, an appeal to her mother for protection; and, a victim of the protective maternal instinct she aroused, I responded. I took her out and dried her. I could not do it if she cried. I wept at my own ineffectuality. Her will to live seemed stronger than my own wish for her death. The cold plunge seemed to have stimulated her sluggish circulation, for she turned a healthy pink and fell into a deep sleep as soon as I changed her.

Miss Fraser had urged me to take Lucy to Dr Morris's baby-clinic, and I knew I had to. And so, one Wednesday afternoon when Lucy was about a month old, I put her in her carry-cot, dressed Julia up warmly, strapped them both in the back of the car and set off. It was the first time I had driven the car for several months, and now it was with some trepidation that I faced the icy roads and the swirling snow. A long tense drive, then a long tense wait. Even Julia sitting quiet and solemnly waiting, no patter, no questions, obviously feeling the intensity of my emotions, without understanding.

At last our name was called. Go in, undress your baby, have her weighed. But, oh God, look at all those other babies—all so plump and stiff with such regular doll-like features. As I undressed Lucy the difference in my baby and those others astonished me. Lucy was so tiny and limp and floppy, her figure rather like that on the refugee poster, with enormous distended abdomen and twig-like limbs. I stared at those other fat rolling babies, and the other mothers stared at Lucy. How I hated those great fat things already seeming to move their arms purposefully, already seeming to take an interest in what was happening to them.

A mother left her naked baby lying on the undressing table where I was tending Lucy, and with a feeling of strong personal hatred towards it I lunged over to push it off. But I did not. Something, God knows what, restrained me, and I stood there, my hands clutching the edge of the table to support myself, just hating it.

And then the nurse called Lucy to be weighed, and all those other mothers looked on while she put my ugly misshapen little Lucy on the scales, and, horror of horrors, what was the nurse saying? 'What did you say your baby weighed at birth Mrs Mussett? Seven-and-a-half pounds? Well I'm afraid she doesn't weigh as much as that now.' And she proceeded to take off weight after weight and click her tongue and shake her head, while everyone looked on. 'No, no, that's all I can make it. Six pounds and one ounce, and you say she's four weeks old? Dear, dear, you'd better come in and see the doctor.' And so we sat down there, Lucy and Julia and me, to wait our turn to see the doctor, and we bowed our heads with shame and stayed quiet.

Dr Morris was quiet and solemn, and tried to be reassuring. 'Oh nothing to worry about Mrs Mussett, these babies are often slow to regain their birth-weight. You need not worry about her heart, the evidence of abnormality is always a bit unreliable, it's a bit early for very definite indications—we'll have to see how she goes. But now we must do something about this feeding—you really must try to get it into her somehow. These babies always are difficult feeders, they need a lot of encouragement.' I tried to protest, to tell him that I had been quite satisfied with the amount of food Lucy took. Julia had always taken only a fraction of the amount prescribed and had thrived on it. By comparison Lucy had a good appetite. But it was useless to protest about that now, with this undeniable evidence before us, that Lucy at a month old weighed much less than when she was born.

Driving home in the premature dusk needed intense concentration. I skidded on icy corners and negotiated the hills carefully. No opportunity to think it all out, to put the pieces of the jig-saw together. What did it mean, this loss of weight? What had he said about her heart? Was I really to be released after all? But I can't think now, I must not think about that now; but already I felt excited with that terrible hope again—perhaps after all Lucy would die a natural death without my having to do anything about it.

How long the minutes seemed waiting for Martin to come home. I put Lucy to bed, tucking her up in the loving way a new mother does when she can afford the luxury of feeling protective towards it. I flitted about the kitchen in a befuddled way, trying to keep my mind on the necessary household chores, getting Julia's tea and preparing the supper. At last the click of the door closing behind him, and trembling violently I tried to tell him about it, but my teeth were chattering so much I bit my tongue, and the words were only an incoherent babble. I collapsed in sobs on his shoulder and Julia cried at his knee. Poor Martin, poor Julia. My extreme emotional reaction to Lucy's condition caused them both a great deal of pain, but I was powerless to control it.

What was it the doctor had said about Lucy's heart? I tried to remember his exact words to repeat to Martin, but I could not.

And what they had meant I was not sure of. Had they meant that there was a possibility that Lucy's heart was defective? What had made him think so? We both scanned the clinic card he had given me. What did those initials on the back mean? We could make no sense of it, and I decided that I had to know more, to have more hard information about mongols, to find out some fact which might confirm my hope that she would indeed die an early natural death.

I went to the reference library the next morning and scanned through every medical book I could find for references to mongolism. There were very few. And the sense of guilt at my purpose made me afraid even to be seen studying the subject. So I left after a while, having made a few relevant but not particularly illuminating notes, and went upstairs to the lending library. There I came upon a book on genetics which stated a hard fact that excited my hope again. 'Fifty per cent of all mongol babies die in the first year of life.' I could not believe it. I checked the date that the book was published: 1957. Surely antibiotics were well established by then. I had read previously that mongols had little resistance to infection, that earlier most had died in early childhood, that only a small percentage survived to the age of puberty; but with modern medical care and antibiotics, these infections were overcome and they survived. Which view was right? Was that one hard statistic still true today?

In the following weeks I spent quite a lot of time searching for information to feed my hope. I discovered that in babies failure to gain weight could be a symptom of a defective heart, but when I questioned the doctor he said that there was no evidence that Lucy's heart might be defective. But we took comfort nevertheless from that one statistic I had found: fifty per cent die in the first year of life—one of every two. Surely ours would be that one. I took comfort in the fact that she still failed to gain weight in spite of adequate feeding. I took comfort in the little blue shadows that came around her mouth, and the way her head continued to loll as the weeks went by.

And as time went by we realized that we would have to tell people. Acquaintances met in the street or the clinic, friends who called, Martin's associates. It took tremendous courage. One braced oneself, and with great effort blurted it out interrupting the exchanged inanities. Too often, in fact I think in every single instance, the statement so cruelly dragged from one was met with a stiffening of the face and after only a moment's hesitation, the slot-machine platitudes of hope. 'It's amazing what they can do nowadays.' 'Oh, you can't be sure, doctors are often wrong aren't they?' 'Oh, my sister's niece had a spastic and he's doing wonders now—ever so happy.' Either that, or it was passed over like a casual remark about the weather. 'Oh, really? Bob's wife had an accident last week. Had to have three stitches.' These reactions left me limp and appalled. It would have given me such satisfaction then if someone had responded by saying 'My God how dreadful!'—but no one did.

And eventually we had to write to our distant friends, 'Our baby is a mongol. . . . We have read that mortality of these babies is very high—as many as 50 per cent die in the first year of life. We live in desperate hope that our dear little Lucy will be among those whose lives are so mercifully brief.' We felt bound to state this at the outset, partly to soften the blow, and because we could no longer bear to hear the falsely hopeful note in other people's voices. And as the weeks went by I loved and cherished the living Lucy, while continuing to hope for her death.

Miss Fraser called every Monday and Friday and Dr Morris insisted that I take Lucy every Wednesday to his baby-clinic. Our hill was ice-packed—a narrow tunnel through the ice-banks built up by the snow-plough. Often it was snowing or blowing a gale or both, and the three-mile drive in the premature dusk was a nightmare. It was the only time in the week that I dared to drive out, but I felt compelled to obey Dr Morris. I was so confused and guilt-ridden that even failing to get her to that clinic had become in my mind a criminal act. I felt as powerless a victim of the National Health Service as any African tribesman of his witch-doctor. The machinery seemed intent on using all its resources to preserve my little Lucy whom Nature and I knew ought to die.

So we went; and always Julia stayed out in the car, sensing the tension of the situation and my own recoiling as yet again the nurse clucked over Lucy's weight or the doctor gave his little homily. Julia could not bear it and preferred to stay alone in the dark cold car and wait, perhaps an hour-and-a-half—waiting, cold, ignored, her personality wilting a little each time. Both Dr Morris and Miss Fraser were constantly advising me about Lucy's feeding. They suggested this or that amount and in vain I protested that indeed she was already taking more than that.

Lucy continued to take milk in greater and greater quantities and I began to suspect that she was suffering from over-feeding rather than under. I wondered whether Dr Morris thought I was trying to starve Lucy, but that would have been quite abhorrent to me. I could not hurt or deprive her. I wanted her death but I could not cause her any pain or suffering. And besides I was greedy for the satisfaction I got from feeding her. I was not so unnatural a mother as not to enjoy that, or to enjoy tending that frail little body, bathing and powdering and dressing her in warm wool, and she smelling so sweet and baby-like.

And at last when Lucy was just over three months old, there came one Wednesday when she did gain weight, and the next and the next. By four months she had regained her birth-weight and Dr Morris said that the crisis was over.

Chapter 5

SPRING HAD COME late after the Big Freeze, and it seemed an eternity since we had left the house except to visit the doctor or get the most urgent shopping. For weeks Julia had been demanding 'Tell me about the spring Mummy'. And I had told her about the primroses and cowslips which would appear in the fields we saw from our windows, and of the blue-tits which would surely again nest in the box as they had for many years now. I told her we would go to the bluebell woods and take a picnic—and as I gave her this romantic picture I found release in it myself, and always in the recesses of my mind was the assumption that by the time that this spring came Lucy would be dead.

But spring at last came and Lucy lived. We packed the rugs and the picnic things and went to the woods. Lucy's head still lolled, but Martin was tall and large, and tucked into the crook of his arm, her head supported on his shoulder, Lucy had a lovely view of the new world. I liked to think she enjoyed those outings. Though she was generally quite passive taking no notice of anything, neither crying nor smiling, yet as she was carried through the woods on her high perch, her little eyes goggled as each new branch passed by—goggled at the tracery of bright green leaves; and when at last Martin put her down in her carry-cot to pick anemones with Julia, she continued to gaze fixedly at the stirring leaves and branches above her head. I cut some large branches of chestnut to stand in an earthen crock beside her cot at home, and she seemed to take quiet pleasure in it. I was indulging myself again. Finding joy in making her little life as rich and pleasurable as possible—anticipating that it would soon be over.

Miss Fraser was constantly trying to persuade me to go to

the local meetings of the Society for Mentally Handicapped Children, and eventually I gave in. The theory is that it helps to meet other people facing the same sort of problem as oneself. I'm afraid it did not work that way with me. Realizing the vast numbers sharing this fate only multiplied the suffering, and facing the same problem did not necessarily mean experiencing the same sort of hell. I felt as alien there as anywhere. But I did meet a friendly woman, Ann Rowlands, who had a mongol boy, Andrew, just two months older than Lucy. She seemed a placid matter-of-fact person, and I envied the way she appeared to be taking this tragedy in her stride. She had three much older children all now at grammar school or university and I thought this must help her to accept Andrew. At least they were well-established personalities who were not likely to be greatly affected by the presence of Andrew, as younger children might be. She asked me to tea and I agreed to go.

I left Julia with Martin on his next off-duty afternoon and took Lucy up to Ann Rowlands. I was as astonished at seeing Andrew as she was at Lucy. Andrew was large and plump, and at seven months sitting sturdily in his chair. Lucy seemed like a limp rag doll beside him. And soon Ann Rowlands was astonishing me even more, 'Yes, one must not say it openly of course, but really it would be a great blessing if they died.' She told me that before her marriage she had been a psychiatric social worker and had often had to deal with mentally-handicapped adults and their families under stress and unable to cope any longer with their child at home. Often it was impossible to find a suitable place in an institution, and when it was, they could not bear the heart-break of parting. She said that she was determined not to let that situation arise with Andrew and had already applied for a place for him in an institution from the age of two. I felt subdued by her objectivity and efficiency.

We settled to tea, Andrew in his high-chair being fed from a spoon and then sucking on a rusk, Lucy passive in her cot, her head still lolling back when she was picked up. Ann went on, 'Have you heard that a lot of these children die in babyhood?' I told her I had and quoted the statistic I had found: one in every two. And we both looked at the babies side by side, and both thought the same thought—which one of these two? We looked long and intently and noted the contrast between them—Lucy limp and frail, tiny and passive, Andrew large and strong, noisy and active. I felt there could be no doubt about which it must surely be. Mrs Rowlands spoke first, 'I pray to God every night to take my Andrew to Him, but it looks as if He is more likely to take your Lucy.'

I saw her again a few times, but within a month of our first meeting, Andrew was dead. We sent spring flowers to the funeral and wept for ourselves.

After Andrew's death I became agitated again. The intense passionate urgency I had felt in the early months had waned a little and I had lapsed into the indulgence of caring for her lovingly, anticipating an early natural death. But now I became afraid again, afraid that in spite of her apparent frailty Lucy would live. Meeting Mrs Rowlands and learning that at least one other apparently normal mother wished her child dead made me—what weakness—bold enough to think that I might find, if not an active collaborator, at least someone to whom I could talk freely about my intentions and find moral support. I remembered Joanne, a friend of many years standing, a successful novelist and playwright. I had seen little of her in the past year though we continued to send spasmodic letters. I wrote immediately asking if we could meet, and, because of the great distance between our homes, suggested meeting in an old historic city about halfway.

Martin and Julia came too. I had not the courage to tell Martin just why I wanted to see Joanne, but he understood that I wanted an opportunity to talk to her, so he planned to take Julia off to the fair on the common, while Joanne and I talked, Lucy with us. We met, and Martin and Julia left us. I can remember now the tremendous sense of occasion I had. This was to be a discussion which, I hoped, would confirm the rightness of my views. I knew that Joanne would think out a moral code for herself, would re-examine the traditional response without prejudice. And so I looked for her support. We talked, or rather

I talked, she mostly sat very quiet, playing idly with Lucy on her lap. She said she would like to think the matter out and then write to me.

We met Martin and Julia in the tea-shop, Julia delighted at meeting her godmother again and Joanne delighted with the three-year-old Julia, who prattled her way through tea, impressing Joanne with her wide vocabulary and knowledge of the city, complimenting the waitress on the cream cakes and telling her she would come again. When Joanne remarked on Julia's vivacity I realized how rare it was nowadays for her to be so. The afternoon out with Martin, meeting her godmother again, Mummy relaxed and apparently happy, all this had combined to excite her and reveal again the lively, curious, loquacious, and happy personality she used to be. Recently she had been much more quiet, even solemn, and sometimes she cried quietly to herself though she could never tell me why.

I waited eagerly for Joanne's letter, never doubting that she would support my views though she might veto my taking action. When her letter came, four or five pages long, I read and re-read and then read it again, stunned. I wish now that I had not destroyed the letter. I cannot remember what it said, only that in two or three pages of reasoned argument she found some purpose in Lucy's life, and in another two or three she urged me strongly—even vehemently—not to take the action I planned, for fear of the consequences to all of us. She spoke of the impossibility of my doing anything to Lucy which would not be detected, and of the pain that would follow for Martin if I were charged with murder or manslaughter, and of the awful effect upon Julia if I were removed from her.

Looking back now I suppose it was sensible advice she gave me, but that judgement has come to me only now, as I write it ten years later. I suppose she must have performed mental gymnastics trying to give me some reason to let Lucy live. But then I only felt betrayed. I felt I had lost my last link with rational and responsible humanity. I felt utterly isolated. Julia was demanding attention and Lucy needed her bath, but I neglected them both to brood over my letter. I was so worried about the evidence of the letter itself that I was in a quandary to know what to do with it. I wanted to keep the letter, I wanted to read it again at some later time—and I searched the house for a suitable hiding place.

Inside a book cover seemed the most anonymous place—so many books, who would ever find that one—but every book I picked up seemed to be one that Martin or some unexpected visitor might select to browse through. I put it inside *Seven Pillars of Wisdom*—a big fat book—but Martin dipped into that so often. I tried a great tome by Arthur Koestler, and discarded that for the same reason. I tried *The Last Stronghold of Sail* and then gave up. I re-read it again hoping to imprint the words on my memory, and then held it out over the kitchen sink and set a match to the corner of each page.

Perhaps if I had kept it and read it again some days or weeks later I should have been able to accept it. Perhaps after all she had not let me down as completely as I felt then. But then the mere refusal of her support devastated me. I shrank a little more.

I heard from her again a week or so later. Perhaps she was anxious at having no response from me. She urged me to see about getting Lucy into a residential home or institution, giving reasons why she thought that best for Lucy and for us. I burned that letter too. I sent no reply for I could think of nothing to say.

After the meeting with Joanne my confidence ebbed away. All the months of Lucy's life I had been sustained, driven on by my determination that Lucy should die, if not naturally then by my hand. Now, interpreting Joanne's advice as rejection of me— since my feelings about this were such an essential part of me—I felt divorced from all humanity. There seemed little purpose in going on, yet stopping would have taken more determination than I was capable of. I began to cry a good deal, bursting unexpectedly into tears when anyone spoke to me. I was quite unable to carry on a conversation because my teeth chattered whenever I spoke. For a long time I had been feeling dizzy, and I frequently had bruises on my left side from bumping into things. I seemed to have developed a leftward sway so that I could not pass through a door-way without bumping myself.

There came a time when I burst into tears at Miss Fraser, and then at a Wednesday visit to the clinic I could not talk to Dr Morris because of my chattering teeth. Inevitably the helplessness I felt made me burst into tears again.

Miss Fraser called unexpectedly one day when Martin was home. She had come to suggest that we let Lucy go into a hospital temporarily for about a month, to give me a rest and to enable us to go on holiday. The idea was so new that I did not know how to react. I was feeling too low-spirited to have any positive feelings about anything. Martin too was undecided, but Miss Fraser was very persuasive. She said that short-stay hospital care was often arranged for handicapped children to allow their parents to take a holiday, and she pointed out that since Lucy was so passive she would not even be aware of the change. She assured us that Lucy would have the best medical attention always at hand, and could only benefit from such care. She said she would call next day for an answer, when we had had time to think about it.

We did not discuss it after she had gone but turned our attention to the household chores and to amusing Julia who seemed suddenly fretful. Perhaps we both needed time to settle the turmoil that this new suggestion had set up within us. Martin brought up the subject again that evening after Julia was in bed. I could not really talk about it, my thoughts were too incoherent; I only cried again and Martin pulled me to him and held me close and we rocked back and forth on the sofa, and through my own tears I became aware that he was crying too, and I knew that he was feeling as helpless and as hopeless as I. We both despaired.

Miss Fraser called again the next day but we had no answer ready. We were both feeling too low to make positive decisions, but she urged us to accept, and said she had already found a place for Lucy, at a large children's hospital where she would be well looked after and could stay for a month. With a sinking heart I turned and looked at Martin appealing to him for a decision. He said, gentle as always, 'I think, dear, it would be best to let her go.'

We discussed it again that evening, in the short intimate time we had together between Julia's bedtime and our own, and discovered that we had both felt reluctant to let her go for the same reason. Not only that we were worried about her care—conversely against all reason, we both felt that she would not be so well cared for by any as by us—but because making plans for Lucy several weeks ahead meant planning for a living Lucy. It was the first time that we had planned our lives or hers on the assumption that she would still be with us. It was hard to face that reality. Until now we had lived each day with the secret hope, even conviction, that by tomorrow, the weekend, next week, Lucy would have passed away, and we three would be alone together as before, confident and unthreatened. But now we must face the reality as other people saw it, and we huddled close to each other again for comfort, fearful of the future.

And so the day came, a few weeks later, when we packed her little belongings and took her to the big hospital forty miles away. It was a bright sunny day and the hospital grounds were full of flowers. It seemed a bright and happy place from the outside. I left Martin in the gardens with Julia since children were not allowed inside, and took Lucy up to the ward. Cold white tiles everywhere, and glass and corridors and starched nurses. What a cold impersonal place to be leaving my little Lucy. How could I leave her? But how could I not when a brisk sister was ushering me into a cubicle instructing me to put her down and fill in forms. What a traitor I felt, abandoning Lucy there. But she did not even know—her little blank eyes passed unknowingly from my face to that other, and round the walls which she did not even recognize as strange—so why did I worry and fret about leaving her? She would be warm and comfortable and well-fed, and Lucy would never ask more of life.

I went out again passing wards full of noisy handicapped children who all seemed happy and confident in spite of their wheel-chairs or crutches, so why did I feel I had betrayed my little Lucy? In the garden Martin approached me anxiously, and even Julia looked strained. I consciously put on a good face and smiled. I told them what a cosy little room Lucy had, and how I had tucked her up with the floppy doll for company, and how interested the nurses were in her. I tried to assure Julia that Lucy would be very happy there, but she was unconvinced. 'Why can't we take Lucy home with us now, Mummy?'

We drove home again and stopped on the way at a tea-shop. I realized that my anxieties for Lucy were being assuaged. The arguments I had used to reassure Martin and Julia were calming me too. Tonight, I thought, I shall not have to kiss Lucy good-night hoping that she will be dead in the morning. I shall not have to pray to God to take her. Lucy is someone else's responsibility tonight—just for one month I can forget to hope and pray and scheme for her. For one month she is someone else's child.

Chapter 6

So we returned home without Lucy. How strange the house seemed without her—yet how could we possibly miss her presence when she was always so silent and passive? Why should the house seem changed without her? We were alone together again, Martin and Julia and I, as we had not been since before Lucy's birth and I felt strangely free and happy. As the days went by I found I had so much more time to play with Julia, and so much more time to think about her. My thoughts had been so exclusively focused on Lucy that Julia had almost ceased to exist for me. I had prepared her meals and washed her clothes and put her to bed when Martin was not there to do it, but the most essential part of her care, playing with her and talking to her, had been reduced to a minimum. I was too preoccupied with Lucy to think much about Julia. But now that Lucy was away, and my anxieties about her held as it were in abeyance, I could notice Julia.

In the past weeks, with my own emotional state, Julia had become increasingly unhappy. She cried frequently and fretted so much at leaving me that she had to give up the play-group which she had previously attended so confidently. From time to time she ran up temperatures for no apparent reason and sat about lethargically looking worried. Undoubtedly at three years old Julia was a pale and subdued version of the personality she had been at two. I began to see how much Julia was being affected by my withdrawal of interest from her. Was she also being made to feel insecure? Was my own complete absorption with Lucy making her feel that she was unloved? That my own emotional state was affecting her had been only too glaringly apparent, but I had been incapable of doing anything about it. Now I made a renewed effort to give her more attention. I resumed my previous habits of playing with her and talking to her and tried to make her feel that she was loved and that all was well with the world. But she still wanted Martin to put her to bed. In the past few months Martin had been the one to put her to bed, read her a story and give her a cuddle, and as the months went by the bed-putting sessions became longer and longer, but I was too relieved to be free of her chatter to think about the significance of it. Now I realized how much more she was look-ing to Martin for security than to me.

Just a week after Lucy had gone to hospital we left for Devon. Martin had booked us in at the Moorland Hotel, a Trust House in the middle of Dartmoor. It was much more expensive than we could afford, but we were both in such a state that camping or boating was more than we could cope with, and the luxury of attractive and comfortable surroundings with every meal pre-pared and put before one, seemed so necessary to us that it was worth dipping into savings for. As Martin said then and many times afterwards, 'It's only money'. Compared with the heart-ache of having a child like Lucy, money seemed relatively un-important.

But it was well-spent. The hotel was indeed luxurious, the food excellent, and Dartmoor surpassingly beautiful. It always surprises me again to discover how much beauty and physical comfort and good food can do to revitalize a sapped spirit, to soothe a battered ego, to elevate one's image of oneself. It was a period of regeneration for all of us. Every morning we hired a small pony from the hotel stables and took Julia out on a leading rein. She took to the moors with the same ease and assurance as she had taken to the water. She scrambled up the sharp high rocks with the agility of a mountain goat, Martin following more cautiously and clumsily after her. She fed the wild ponies with clumps of purple moor-grass and cheerfully pursued them when they lost interest. She picked whortle-berries and heather and watched butterflies and birds. She endeared herself to every-one with her winning ways and blunt comments on her sur-roundings. On one occasion in the dining-room, accustomed at home to eating from a formica-topped table in the kitchen, she demanded to know why all the tables were covered up with sheets, and on another to know why all the waiters wore the sort of clothes Daddy wore on special occasions in the evening. Didn't they have any others? She enchanted a pair of old ladies by presenting them with a few wilting wild flowers, and her own wilting spirit revived in this relaxed and friendly atmosphere as her flowers did in water. Dressed as always in cotton trousers and T-shirts with her short golden hair in tight angel curls round her head she looked more like a boy than a girl, and was often taken for one. At her command we went in search of running brooks and splashing waterfalls where she paddled and splashed delightedly. Here there was little sign of the silent anxious child who clung to me waiting with Lucy at the doctor's surgery, or screamed in terror at leaving me at the play-group. Here she confidently trotted off across the garden leaving us herself to go and talk to her ageing friends.

For Martin and I too it was an oasis of calm and peace and blissful forgetfulness. We found joy ourselves in seeing Julia so happy again, and her instant delight in every new butterfly or rivulet revived in us a sense of wonder and of communion with Nature and Life. It gave us what we had almost lost—a reason for living—a desire to live. On our very last evening, after Julia had fallen asleep, Martin and I went out on to the moor under the stars. The full moon silhouetted the rocks and bushes, and small mammals stirred the grasses in their flight before us. The very timelessness and changelessness of the scene dwarfed us, and with us, our pains and problems. The scene around us now was much as it had been for the past few thousand years. Nothing had changed; sky, landscape, plants and animals, all were the same then as now—even we. Technical skills and cultural habits had multiplied and accumulated over the years and our lives were socially more complicated because of it—but under the skin, had we changed? We loved our young, protected the weaker members of society, killed to eat, showed aggression to our enemies, then as now: no, we had not changed. The ponies moved stealthily and we found ourselves too walking lightly and talking in whispers, fearful of disturbing that profound peace.

Home again. Another week yet before we fetch Lucy home. We have another week of thinking of ourselves, giving loving attention to Julia, of forgetting about Lucy. So why does my stomach heave as the cold fear grips me again? Fear of what? Fear of what life will do to Lucy, and what Lucy will do to us. Martin too was suddenly grave and sober, Julia curiously silenced. The very walls seemed impregnated with the fears Lucy had engendered. How was she I wondered. Had she been contented? Had she pined for me? Of course not, my common sense told me, she does not know you so how can she miss you? She does nothing but sleep and she is as warm and comfortable there as here. But my fear for her and guilt at leaving her was outside the realm of reason. Was she even alive—perhaps she had died while we were away and they had lost the forwarding address. But of course, common sense told me again, this was not possible —they would have found us somehow. But perhaps she was ill —seriously failing—I must phone to find out how she was. But why had I not phoned before? Three weeks had gone by with no news of her—why ever had I not phoned? Whatever would the hospital think of me, abandoning her so completely? I was overcome with guilt at my negligence, but in fact it was more than that. The intense strain of worrying about Lucy, of looking for her death, of fearing the consequences of her living, of guilt at having brought her into the world and at having inflicted her upon Julia—this was so great that we needed to forget her existence, to rest our minds from being constantly focused on this one aspect of our lives to the exclusion of all else. This indeed was the real value of Lucy's stay in hospital, and given that opportunity our minds rested and turned back to Julia and slowly, to the other pleasures in our lives, to the extent that we did not even think of phoning. We were incapable of directing our thoughts to her for a short time and then away again—if we phoned we would be absorbed, possessed again.

But now I had thought of it, and overcome with guilt I picked up the phone. I heard sister's voice and stammered out an incoherent apology for not having done so before, searching for reasons and excuses, all of them sounding feeble. Sister however, was only waiting for a pause so that she could tell me about Lucy. Lucy had indeed been ill while we were away. She had developed a tummy infection and this had led to pneumonia. They had put her in an oxygen tent and after some days she had rallied. Now, sister assured me, Lucy was quite recovered, so there was no point in rushing up to see her. She was out of danger, although she had lost some weight and was being specially nursed and fed.

Oh my God, what had I done? I should have been with her— I should have nursed her myself. I was swamped with guilt at having left her, just when she needed me most. I was in an emotional turmoil again. And then the implication of what sister had said leapt to my mind. Lucy had had pneumonia. It was what we had hoped and prayed for in the early days, anticipating, after what Dr Morris had said, that she would die of it. But now, when at last the expected happened, she was already in hospital, and it had been promptly diagnosed and treated—so promptly as to save her life. Oh my God, why had I not kept her at home? If she had been at home when it came diagnosis would have been delayed and treatment may well have come too late. It would have been a quick and quiet end to her little life, and to all our heartache, now and in the long years looming ahead of us. Why did I let her go? I had given up hope that God or Nature would release us all—and that had cost us her death. Would I ever forgive myself for that? I had known, I had been sure, in those early days, that she would die—why had I given up, lost my courage and determination? I should have had more faith in my own judgement and Martin's. And now my weakness had let the moment pass, slip by unnoticed. Now she would be forever the albatross around our necks—not just mine, but Martin's and Julia's too.

And yet I longed to see my little Lucy. How illogical. How confused. I was distressed to think of her body emaciated again, and spent the remaining days without her alternately planning extra vitamin drops to build her up and hoping that perhaps even now she might have a relapse from which she would not recover. Instinct drove me, for my own maternal satisfaction, to protect, to nurse, to love her; but the long-term prospect of her living was so awful that reason made me hope for her death. I was possessed again, my attention riveted exclusively on Lucy.

Chapter 7

I AM SURE that Lucy smiled when she saw me. Swathed in pink woollens with pink in her cheeks and streaks of golden silk hair escaping her bonnet, she had never looked prettier. How my heart went out to her. How comforting and right it felt to hold her in my arms again. Yes she was thinner, but yet I detected signs of development. Her head did not loll quite so limply, and her body seemed stiffer to hold. Obviously her muscle-tone was improving. Eight months old now, and my little Lucy really was becoming 'Lucy', a definite personality in her own right, not just an anonymous mongol baby.

Home with her again I began to indulge myself with loving and caring for her, not thinking about the future, but waiting suspended, as if for Fate to decide the issue for us. Julia was happier too, now that I was less distraught, and I encouraged her to help me care for Lucy, bathing and dressing and feeding her, in a way I could not have done before, being too distracted. Julia began to play with her too. She had a sturdy wooden doll's cot which we had bought at the cattle-market auction, and we found that, propped with pillows, we could wedge Lucy into a near-sitting position, and the firm sides of the small cot supported her securely. Thus propped Lucy lolled back contentedly on the pillows, her little round eyes wandering vacantly, while Julia prattled and played around her. 'Come along my pretty one,' she would say when Lucy's mouth fell open and her tongue sagged, 'come along my little baby, we all know what a pretty tongue you've got, showing off again are you?' And getting little response Julia would busy herself building elaborate harvest-festival-like edifices around the cot. She gathered all the vegetables and fruit she could find, potatoes, oranges, onions, and apples, lemons and sprouts and Oxo cubes, all carefully balanced and artistically arranged, and then decorated it further with silver-paper wrappings from chocolate and glass necklaces draped between the fruit, and even sugar lumps or a sprinkling of bright orange lentils. And Lucy sat in the middle still and quiet, 'Like a queen, Mummy,' said Julia. And when she had finished she invited Lucy to see how grand she looked. 'Look, look, little queen, you are the queen of the harvest.' And when she could get no response she would despair, 'Oh why won't she look, Mummy? Why won't she look?'

We continued to take Lucy to the baby-clinic on alternate Wednesday afternoons—and these continued to be anxious occasions for me. I never knew which of four partners I should see, but I felt intimidated by all of them. The repeated advice about feeding, the constant warning to guard her from infection, keep her warm, feed her often, stimulate her—these worried and depressed me greatly. I felt so inadequate. They spoke to me in gentle insistent tones as if I were an idiot myself without an idea at all of how to look after a baby. It was always after these sessions that I began to despair again.

The health visitor still continued to call at least once a week, and she always spoke about feeding, until I could bear it no longer, and screamed out at her, 'If anyone mentions feeding to me again, I'll throw a kettle at his head'. Poor Miss Fraser, she was so surprised. But it was not her that I was really railing against, but the persistence of emphasis that was put upon it, and the doctor's refusal to believe the true facts I gave him—that Lucy was already taking far more milk than he prescribed. No-one, then, suspected that she might have a mal-absorption condition.

But we had begun to expand a little, to live a normal life again. One Sunday in early autumn we set out to spend the day with Martin's mother. Julia was delighted at the thought of seeing Granny again, and it gave me a strange feeling of elation to be doing so ordinary and natural a thing as spending a day with Granny when Lucy was with us. I realized then just how much we had limited our lives, being obsessed with Lucy. We had seen little of relatives or friends since Lucy's birth.

Martin's mother had come once for a day in the spring. Several times we had dissuaded her, using the bad weather as an excuse, but at last we could put her off no longer. When she arrived I was tense and aloof with her, afraid that she would talk about Lucy. I could not bear then to discuss Lucy as if she would live, but did not dare to tell Ma how I wished for her death. It was the same with all our relatives and friends. I felt so alien that I shunned every one of them, and since Lucy's birth our social life had been minimal.

In the following months we slowly began to see our few relatives and friends again, always taking Lucy with us. Soon we began to hear, on all sides it seemed, the suggestion that we should find a home, an institution for Lucy. I cannot remember now when it was that we first began to consider the possibility instead of brushing it aside peremptorily. It came to us slowly and painfully as we began to face the fact that Lucy was going to live.

Was there perhaps, somewhere, a small residential home, bright and cheerful, where Lucy would be well cared for, even loved? Would she be happy away from us? Could we let her live away if we visited her frequently, took her out, brought her home for holidays? Was such a life possible? We discussed it together again and again, going over all the implications we could think of, to Lucy and to us.

I recalled the things I had learned at college about institutionalized babies, and re-read my notes on Bowlby's classic on the subject. That was pretty damning—but surely the effects on a mentally-handicapped child, one as grossly handicapped as Lucy, could not be similar. And I knew from first hand the effects of keeping such a child in the family. How did one weigh that in the balance? Martin urged me to discuss it with the doctor, and reluctantly I agreed.

When the time came I waited even more anxiously than usual, my hands clammy with perspiration, my voice shrill as I rebuked Julia for fidgeting. And then I learned that the doctor on duty that day was the one I found most unsympathetic, so I lost my courage and decided to wait till the next visit.

At the next baby-clinic Julia sat beside me whimpering with earache. It was a long wait that afternoon, and as time went by the whimper became a cry, and she writhed about with the pain, and was so hot and flushed that she was obviously running a temperature. It became clear that I could not continue to sit and wait with her any longer, so I went to the secretary and explained that I could not wait to take Lucy into the doctor, but would bring her next week. It did not even occur to me to ask the doctor to see Julia. No-one had shown the slightest interest in Julia's health or development since Lucy had arrived, and in my highly suggestible state I had adopted their attitude. I was surprised therefore when I found the secretary following me out to say that the doctor would see Julia. He found that she had an abscess in her ear and a raised temperature. He prescribed an antibiotic and a sedative and told me to get her home to bed. He did not even mention Lucy. I was astonished. He even told me not to bother to bring Lucy next week as Julia would still need to be kept indoors. Once again I was struck with remorse at my neglect of Julia—and I burned with resentment at the heavy emphasis everyone put on every slight aspect of Lucy's health and development while not bothering at all about Julia's, until this extreme condition arose.

And so it was some time before I was able to discuss Lucy's future with my doctor. In the intervening weeks Martin and I had examined and re-examined all the possibilities, growing daily more anguished, changing our minds repeatedly and beset by doubts about any future for Lucy. I wished that I could talk to Dr Morris about it, but he had left the practice. His place had been taken by Dr Baker, a conscientious doctor who had once been a missionary. He had always spent a lot of time with Lucy, and a lot of time talking to me about her, even though it was only to reiterate instructions for her care he had given me twenty times before.

Summoning all my courage I spoke to him about the possibility of a home for her. He gave me his opinion, in the same quiet insistent voice he always used, that he was sure that all handicapped children should live at home with their families. He said he did not believe in separating such children from the community. He was sure this was best for Lucy—she would get on just as well at home as away, and after all weren't all children the responsibility of their parents? Did I know how much it cost to keep a child in an institution? He assured me that although Lucy was severely retarded, as she grew older she would fit into the family quite well—being only a little different from my other child. I felt too subdued, too crushed to answer. What did he mean by that last statement? Useless to point out that at Lucy's age, eleven months, Julia had been walking, that she was talking volubly at eighteen months, and now at three-and-a-half was already beginning to read. What did he mean? I busied myself adjusting Lucy's clothing, gathered up Julia, and slunk away, ashamed.

Oddly enough it was Miss Fraser who, at her next visit broached the subject. She asked if we had thought about Lucy's future, so I told her about my conversation with Dr Baker and she was very puzzled by his response. She questioned me then about how Martin and I felt about it, how we viewed the prospect of keeping her at home, whether we had considered the effect on Julia, if we knew anything about the homes in our county. I told her everything we had considered, and of our hope that a small pleasant loving home could be found for her, and of my fears lest she suffer any deprivation because of it.

Miss Fraser stayed over an hour listening sympathetically to me, and pointing out herself some aspects we had missed. She said that she did not have any fixed views about it because every case she met had different factors to be considered. An important one, she said, was the degree of handicap. In Lucy's case this looked clear-cut—she was severely retarded and would probably only develop to a very limited degree, not enough to form fixed personal relationships with a particular individual, not enough to be able to recall a face or a place that was not immediately present, not enough to feel home-sickness or fear. She said that Lucy would need always to be kept warm, to be carefully fed, to be treated kindly—but with such treatment she would always be happy. She told me I could forget the findings of Bowlby;

since Lucy's perceptions were so limited she would not suffer the same mental and emotional deprivations as normal children; and, besides, in the particular home she had in mind for Lucy, conditions were very different from those in the institutions Bowlby studied. Surprised and eager I asked her more about the 'particular home' she had in mind.

She told me then of a small home about fifteen miles away, which had belonged to the Invalid Children's Aid Association before being taken over by the National Health Service. It was a large old house with a lovely garden. There was accommodation for 25 babies under five, and, counting the kitchen staff and gardener as well as nurses, there were 28 staff. She urged me to go along to see it, and said that she could arrange it; but that first I must speak to Dr Baker again, since he was the one who must recommend Lucy for a place before there was any possibility of her going there.

She came again in the evening to talk to Martin about it. She told him that she thought it best for Lucy to go away. The time would come, she said, when Lucy would have to go to an institution, and she herself thought it was easier on everyone if she went early—before the break became too great a wrench for all of us. She thought too that it was best for Julia—since she was an only sibling and an older girl. And last, she said, she thought it was best for me. With my long medical history she did not think I was robust enough to cope with Lucy over the coming years—either physically or emotionally.

Martin was quiet and grave for a long time after she had gone, and I was quiet too. I sat quietly mending while Martin puffed his pipe, slouched deep in the armchair gazing into the fire. He finished his pipe and knocked it out on the grate, and I put down my sewing. We looked at each other then, and he held out his arms to me. He hugged me close and we rocked together in silence. And then he said, his voice muffled against my hair, 'You know what we must do, love? We must move heaven and earth to get Lucy into the home that Miss Fraser talks about. It's the only thing to do.'

And so it was decided that I should bring up the subject again with Dr Baker. Miss Fraser had impressed upon me the need to let him know quite definitely how we both felt about it, and to tell him too of our reasons. And so Martin and I rehearsed together the arguments to support our decision, and to clarify it in my own mind I wrote it down. I would tell him about my own experience while teaching handicapped children. Most of the children I had met in residential special schools had been happy children: they were in a sheltered community with others like themselves, where to have that affliction was to be usual and accepted and a full member of that society. Only the whole would have felt alien. The real hurt for these children came when they were sixteen, and left their protected environment to live in the unthinking, uncaring world, where people resisted relating to someone so different from themselves. This was the real problem for many handicapped children—but it would not concern Lucy. Lucy would obviously stay in a home for the rest of her life. I would tell him too of my own sister, and of how my mother's total preoccupation with her handicap adversely affected us all—and even in the end, Melanie herself.

We debated whether it would be a good idea for Martin to come with me, but were doubtful about it, and since there was also the problem of leaving an unhappy Julia somewhere, we decided against it, but planned that Martin should be at home at that time to look after Julia.

Dr Baker looked rather surprised when I brought up the subject for a second time. I started to tell him that Martin and I felt that it might be best for Lucy to go away—and instantly he began to reiterate his own views exactly as he had done before. I started to expand on our reasons, but he was hardly interested; he simply said that on this point we must agree to differ. He seemed to be treating it as a purely rhetorical argument, seeming not to see that we had the right, even the duty, to act upon our own judgement.

I pressed more urgently saying that at least we wanted to take the next step, to have our case put before the county medical officer, but he was adamant. He had, he said, to act in accordance with his own conscience, and he would not recommend that any handicapped child should leave home—unless it needed hospital treatment. 'After all', he said, 'you are not the only one. I have child-patients who are spastic or crippled or deaf, they are just as bad as yours you know.' 'As bad,' I cried, suddenly roused to indignation, 'you think they are as bad? They are infinitely worse. They will be expected, or will want, to fit into the world when they grow up—and will be only too conscious then of their handicap, their difference, their unlovableness. My God they are infinitely worse off than Lucy. She will always be protected by her limited awareness. She will not even know there is an outside world—she will not know that she is different.' I paused, but Dr Baker remained silent, seeming stunned by my outburst. 'I know that handicapped children of normal intelligence are far worse off,' I went on, 'and I thank God that Lucy is not one of them. But Lucy is my responsibility—as you said—she is the one I must concern myself with and make provision for.' He was silent for awhile, but unbending. 'Well, that is your concern,' he said, dismissing me.

And so it was all to come to nothing. All that heart-searching, worry, fretting, and turmoil—it had all been in vain. Miss Fraser had made it quite clear that nothing could be done without our doctor's sanction. Lucy's future and ours was to be dictated by our doctor's viewpoint—we were to have nothing at all to do with the decision. We were victims of a system that gave a GP the power of a god.

Despair enveloped us then. We had been a whole and complete family unit before Lucy's birth. The future rolled out before us deep and rich, full of promise. Why had we put that in jeopardy by deliberately, intentionally, seeking another baby? Our own greed for life had been our undoing. Why had we not been content with what we had? All my life I had lived as if each day was only a preparation for tomorrow. Now there just did not seem to be a tomorrow—not one which I could bear to contemplate.

And then resentment welled up in me when I remembered what Dr Baker had said; Lucy was my responsibility—my responsibility—my responsibility. The words echoed in my head against a background of ironic laughter. My responsibility, when my own response to her condition, a natural and a reasoned response—to kill her—had been so effectively thwarted by society's laws? Whose responsibility did that make her? In the heat of my anger I railed in my note-book:

> You, society at large, have condemned my daughter to life. I would have killed her then, when they told me she was a mongol. Urged by the vehement instinct of a mother to protect her young, I would have killed to protect her from a harsh unfriendly world where she would be a stranger always and everywhere. Prompted by love, by pity, by compassion, I would have killed her then. It is you, remote society, who uphold unquestioningly your rigid law—Thou shalt not kill—even for mercy. If she had been my responsibility—mine only—she would have been sleeping at peace now in the quiet village churchyard, with winter-jasmine coming into bloom upon her grave and the last rose-bud shrivelled with frost. Oh that she had been exclusively my responsibility! You—society at large—have condemned my daughter to life, and in so doing have made her your responsibility, not mine: what are you going to do about her now.

But society it seemed did not feel moved to do anything about her. Even Miss Fraser did not call for many days, and when she did come she could hold out no hope. She too had seen Dr Baker, with the same result. There seemed little that we could do. We discussed a few possible lines with Miss Fraser, but they all seemed hopeless—and in our low spirits we gave up before we started. Suddenly Martin announced that he was going to see Dr Baker himself, but he came back looking even more harassed than when he went. Dr Baker had told him that the possibility of a place in a home was, in any case, quite hopeless, since there were so many more patients than places. There was a two-year waiting period for those on the list, but one's home conditions had to be very unsatisfactory before one got on to it. And even then, he pointed out, there was no chance of Lucy going to

Beechwood House, the small home for 25—that was only for very special patients. No, Lucy, if she should ever be offered a place which was unlikely, would be sent to Haughton, a vast Victorian institution for mentally handicapped and mentally disturbed alike—for 1500 of them. 'It will provide adequate custodial care,' he had said, 'if that is what you want.'

That was unthinkable—quite unthinkable. The idea filled us with abhorrence, and would very effectively have stopped us from taking any further action. But Miss Fraser was not so easily put down. She called unexpectedly a few days later to say that she had been in touch with the county medical officer, and had arranged for a county psychologist to come down to see Lucy. I learned later that Miss Fraser had risked a reprimand herself for her direct approach to the county without Dr Baker's authority. The psychologist would be coming the very next day, and the possibility of a place for Lucy would depend upon her report. I pointed out the bleak picture that Dr Baker had drawn —long waiting lists, Haughton—but Miss Fraser begged me not to be too depressed by that, to wait and see what the psychologist, Miss Mason, advised.

Again the tense waiting. I wished that Martin had been home that day—but the nature of his work made that impossible. I washed and dressed Lucy with trembling fingers, changed her again and fetched her carry-cot down, all the time trying to suppress Julia because I was too anxious to attend to her chatter. I waited for the swish of tyres in the courtyard, and then picked Lucy up again and stood looking out of the window, expecting every car on the hill to be Miss Mason's. She was young, disconcertingly young. How could anyone so young make the decisions Martin and I had been grappling with for months? She opened her caseful of tricks, and seeing Julia's interest, showed her one or two of the psychological toys she had. That was kind of her; it gave me time to compose myself.

I propped Lucy in an armchair well padded out with cushions and Miss Mason asked me about her. Yes, Lucy was eleven months old now; yes, she was still on a completely liquid diet; no, she could not sit alone yet, but proudly I pointed out the two

3

teeth she had produced at ten months. Miss Mason took Lucy then and laid her down upon the floor where she lay inert. Miss Mason turned her over on to her face carefully placing her hands palm downwards on a level with her head, but Lucy only moved her head slightly sideways so that her face was not flat on the carpet, she did not raise her head. We propped her up again and Miss Mason gave her a block to hold, but it fell from her limp fingers. She gave her a rod, and this Lucy grasped; she held up a bright bauble but had difficulty persuading Lucy to focus her eyes on it before she moved it across her range of vision, and Lucy followed its course for only a moment. She had a number of other things which piled up or fitted together in some way, but they served only to amuse Julia. She told me then what she thought the future would be for Lucy. She would, she said, develop slowly, but would probably never exceed a mental age of about two years. She would probably learn to feed herself and to walk, perhaps to wash and dress herself with help. But she was unlikely to develop speech at all, or at best she might achieve a vocabulary of half-a-dozen words, and may never develop real bowel or bladder control.

She asked me then what we had in mind for the future, and I told her how we felt. She told me that the current feeling about such children was that they should remain at home with their families in a normal environment, not shut away where society never saw them. How else, she said, would society learn to accept them? So the new policy was to leave them with their families— 'Community Care' they called it. Bitterly I said that I had not noticed that my community cared—didn't she mean family care? I hadn't noticed either that the community cared much about any handicapped people. While some might tolerate a handicapped child, there was little evidence that the average community— even an intelligent and enlightened community—cared much for handicapped adults.

I could not see, I told her, that the community did care, and that being the case, I did not see how one could bring it about by legislation. True, there were a number of small groups of voluntary and social workers who cared very much, and did what they could in fund-raising, in providing services and even in visiting, but what really mattered to the person concerned, was not the attitude of the occasional visitor—but that of his neighbour, his colleague, and the people he met in the ordinary course of his daily life. To force the handicapped child to stay in a hostile environment would not change society—it would only hurt the handicapped. It must be society which changes its attitude to the handicapped—since the handicapped cannot function as does society. That change must come first, and until it does, how can you deny shelter to those who seek it?

I asked what effect the community-care policy had on the families involved, but she said it was too early to know, not much work had been done on that. And then, like Dr Baker, she took refuge in quoting costs—the vast sums the county was spending to support the mentally handicapped already in their institutions. At that I quite lost my control again. 'It's a pity,' I said heatedly, 'if society cannot afford to care for these children, that she does not allow them an easy death as soon as they are born. Euthanasia would solve most of your problems and mine.' She remained silent and looked abashed, and I felt sorry for my outburst. After all she was very young and inexperienced. It was unlikely that she had had so much opportunity as I to observe and identify with the handicapped. I could not blame her for not sharing my viewpoint. I apologized, and offered her coffee which to my surprise she accepted.

While I made coffee in the kitchen she played on the floor with Julia and her box of tricks. 'It's a very bright child you have here,' she said, referring to Julia. I was comforted by that and warmed to her. Before she left she said that she would do what she could to get Lucy a place at Beechwood House, since that was what we wished, but the pressure on places was very great and she was not too hopeful.

I was elated then—quite elated. I desperately wanted someone to talk to, to tell about it. There was after all a possibility that Lucy might go to Beechwood. And the possibility became, in my unstable frame of mind, a certainty. I just had to tell someone, but there was no-one there to tell. Unable to contain myself any longer, I told Julia. I told her that Lucy was going away to live in a small home especially for babies like herself—slow-growing babies—babies who did not want to run about and talk and play as she did, but who spent all their time in bed being looked after by nurses. On sunny days, I said, they would have their cots pushed out into the beautiful garden so that they could look at the bright flowers, see the trees move in the wind, and watch the birds come and go. Lucy would not really grow up, I told Julia, as she would. Lucy would stay a baby for a very long time, so it was best for her to go away. We would go to see her often, and would take her on outings with us just as before. And then my control broke, and I laughed hysterically till laughter changed to tears, and I could not stop till I saw that I had frightened Julia so much that she was crying too.

I should not have told Julia then, and like that, when I was in such an emotional state. To involve a child so young was unforgivable of me. I know it now and I knew it then, but I was intoxicated with relief and quite unable to control myself. But when I saw Julia crying it shocked me into sobriety. 'My God,' I thought, 'what am I doing to this child? I must take hold of myself.'

I did what I could to soothe and reassure Julia, and got her some ice-cream and chocolate sauce, and feeling in need of a reviver myself, made a pot of tea. I remembered my grandmother's favourite remedy for all ills—and added a little whisky to my tea. I had enough tea and whisky and aspirins to tranquillize me into an emotional void, and played games with Julia and read her stories till Martin came home and I could tell him about it.

At last he arrived, and I related the conversation with Miss Mason as exactly as I could remember it. He listened, calm and patient as always, and then reminded me that Miss Mason had made no promises. Beechwood was only a possibility, not a certainty, not even a probability. But still the mere fact that Miss Mason had listened to our reasons, had taken our own wishes into consideration, would perhaps put Lucy on some sort of waiting-list for a place in the future, all these made us feel

suddenly confident and hopeful. There was now a possibility of
an acceptable future for a living Lucy, and we ourselves were
able to influence it.

And so we felt more hopeful that night than we had for a long
time. Martin took Julia up to bed and read her a story while I
prepared our supper. We liked to have our meal together after
she was in bed. It was a quiet and intimate time for us, a time
when we could commune without interruption or distraction.
We drew comfort and strength from our quiet time together.
And so we shared our supper from a trolley by the fire, and
Martin put on some of our favourite records—operatic arias,
folk-songs, sea-shanties. When it was finished he drew me to
him on the sofa and we clung together in silence. He kissed me,
softly at first, on my cheeks, my eyes, my hair, and then more
hungrily and passionately, and I returned his passion. He held
my face between his two hands and looked at me tenderly.
'Shall we go to bed, love?' he said. I knew what he meant. Since
Lucy's birth we had shared our double-bed as before, and as
before we had held each other close, but, unlike before, we had
not gone beyond that. The shock of having given birth to Lucy
had been so great for both of us that we dared not have inter-
course again—we dared not take the risk. We had tried once or
twice, when Lucy had been a few months old, using a multiplicity of contraceptive methods, but we were so anxious that
we could never put our faith in them, and our loving was clumsy
and unsuccessful, so we had turned away from it altogether. But
now we went up to bed and clung to each other again, and
Martin was gentle and tender and I found myself responding
to his caresses, and it was all right again.

Chapter 8

JULIA WAS ALREADY trotting into our room when we awoke next morning. It was a bright windy day, with a high blue sky and watery sunshine, fluffy cumulus clouds scudding fast across the sky. It was a day off for Martin, and seeing the fine weather he said, 'Shall we go out today?' 'An outing?' responded Julia, excitedly. 'Shall we go on an outing?' I realized then how few 'outings' we had had since Lucy had been born. Family activities had been restricted and festive occasions rare. But now my eyes caught Martin's over Julia's tousled curly head and we smiled at each other. Yes, it was time for an outing.

We decided to go into the cathedral city twenty or so miles away, driving by an indirect route which would take us through extensive woodland. If the sun was still shining we would stop and picnic. Julia was happy again. She chattered and babbled away to herself as she packed what she thought she would need; Wellingtons, plastic mac, hairbrush, teddy, and of course, Hip and Lock. Hip was a hippopotamus, a sculptured model about three inches long, and Lock was his baby. They came with us wherever we went and with them came their necessities: a woollen rug in case it turned cold, a handkerchief—'To wipe Lock's eyes if he cries, Mummy'—and lunch, today a single raisin and a few biscuit crumbs wrapped in a square inch of tissue paper. When Julia had finished her packing and we ours, she dressed herself in the tweed coat I had made for her and got Daddy to fasten her string of beads on top, 'So everyone can see them, Daddy'.

Joyously we set off, each of us buoyed up by the happy family mood—stimulated by the anticipation of an interesting day out. Only Lucy remained her usual placid self. She suffered us to put on her coat and bonnet and blankets without complaint, and,

secure in her carry-cot, allowed us to strap it down in the car
without response. It was bright and cold in the woods. Our
cheeks reddened as we ran to keep warm, leaving Lucy parked
in the car for awhile. We climbed on some logs, and Martin
swung Julia on a drooping branch. It was good to see them
playing together again—Julia laughing, Martin smiling his
lovely relaxed smile.

We went for a walk along the dry bridle path, starting the
occasional pheasant as we went, Martin carrying Lucy and I the
picnic basket. Julia, compulsive gatherer, still found enough
withered bracken, coloured leaves, rose-hips and bluebell seed-
pods to make an interesting posy. It began to rain so we took
shelter in a small open-fronted coop, used in the spring for
rearing young pheasants. It was just high enough for Martin to
sit with the roof brushing his hair. We had our picnic there, hot
soup, chicken-legs, French bread and fruit-cake, while we
waited for the rain to stop. Julia looked out excitedly, watching
rain-drops explode as they landed on the shiny holly leaves, or
seep stealthily into the soft mud. Well-protected she went outside laughing as she stomped about in the mud, making puddles
of her foot-marks. The rain stopped before long, and we were
able to get back to the car comparatively dry.

In the city we put Lucy's carry-cot in the wheeled-trundler,
and set off for the cathedral. We walked around the age-old
ruins and cloisters, where we had walked so often before, where
we had brought Julia when she too was in the carry-cot and
trundler—the same one. Strange to think how inanimate
possessions shared our experiences and formed a time-bridge
between them. We little thought then, when we brought Julia in
the trundler, that we would come again with another baby, or
dreamed that she would be a Lucy—with all the pain and
anguish that that had caused. Strange that we should have
experienced that and then come here again to the same spot as
we had brought Julia. What might happen to us before we came
here again? What impression did we leave behind on the
impregnable walls—of our visit with Julia? with Lucy? I
remembered a particular visit with Julia when she was about two

months old, and on that occasion too it was raining. We stopped in the cloisters and sat on a low wall to give Julia a bottle. She was always a reluctant feeder, but here she drank a whole bottle straight down, for the first and probably the only time in her life. Lucy now did the same thing—though she was eleven months old and for her whole bottles were usual.

We left the cathedral to look at the shops. Martin and Julia spent some time in the pet-shop watching the antics of the mice and monkeys, the rabbits and the puppies, and they bought food to feed the birds in the square.

We arrived home to find a note in the letter-box. Miss Fraser had called while we were out, and would call again the next day. Immediately we were filled with apprehension. Why had she called again so soon? What news had she brought? We were sobered again, and quietly we put Julia and Lucy to bed, had our supper, and retired early ourselves, vaguely troubled.

Martin was home next morning when Miss Fraser called again. She said that Miss Mason had recommended that Lucy be admitted to Beechwood, and that she be given the next vacancy. Martin asked her when that would be. She could not be sure but thought that it might be 'quite soon'. Martin asked if we could visit Beechwood and meet the matron, and Miss Fraser said she would arrange it.

When she had gone Martin and I clung to each other saying nothing. I was feeling very frightened and Martin understood it —perhaps he was feeling the same way. 'It's going to be all right, love, it's going to be all right,' he whispered fiercely in my hair. I was glad Martin was there. Miss Fraser had brought us good news, we should have been glad and relieved; it was what we had wanted, or at least, it was what we had decided was best. But we did not feel glad, only uneasy and vaguely frightened, and overawed at the responsibility of the action we were taking.

When we visited Beechwood we saw it with very mixed feelings. Remembering it now, after having seen so many homes and schools and institutions for the mentally handicapped, I realize how privileged we were to be offered such an unusually luxurious place—but then we came to it from the comfort of our own home, and compared it with that as a refuge for Lucy. It came out of the comparison very well nevertheless.

It was a large attractive house, standing well back from the road in a large well-groomed garden. Only the board mounted by the gate indicated its difference from the other similar houses surrounding it. But as soon as one was inside, the rather bare clinical furnishings and the faint smell of disinfectant reminded one of its function. Matron came to greet us: young, smiling, confident. She had flowers on the desk in her office and seemed warm and friendly. She took us through the various rooms of the house, each one of them with four or more cots in it. Mostly the children lay inert, much as Lucy did, though many of them were physically as well as mentally handicapped, or with organs malfunctioning. Some had long emaciated limbs and matron explained that they were in fact much older than five, but remained there because there seemed little point in moving them. Their behaviour, and the care they needed, was that of month-old babies. Others had the enlarged heads of hydrocephalous, with drainage tubes in their heads, and another suffering some internal disorder with drainage tubes from the abdomen; and yet another being intravenously fed. Most of them, if not all, would remain bedridden all their lives, unknowing, unheeding, existing only to be fed and cared for. There were toys on most of the cots—cradle-plays strapped across the top, or soft toys tied to the end. Occasionally there was a child sitting pillow-propped in his cot, actually grasping or playing with his toys—but mostly they lay back gazing vacantly into space. I began to protest to matron that Lucy was not handicapped physically, was not suffering any organic disorder, but matron quickly reassured me, as we went from room to room, that there were others like my Lucy, who were together downstairs. She said the county liked to send her a few such, because if all the patients were of the severely affected, completely unresponsive type, the work was most depressing for the nurses, since they got no 'feed-back' in response to their efforts. A few little mongols, who were usually so happy and mischievous, enlivened the scene, and added interest to the otherwise unrewarding task of caring for those much more severely afflicted. For the first time I had the idea that my little Lucy might have a rôle to play, and it was here. But it was only a glimmer of justification for her life: how much better I thought, if all these babies had been allowed the mercy of an easy death. The nurses seemed kindly, the rooms clean and bright, it was warm and comfortable. Obviously the babies were given every possible care—but yet we both had the feeling that the exercise was purposeless and futile.

We saw four or five little mongols when we came to the playroom, all looking, as they do, like each other's twin. They were playing on the warm cork-tiled floor with a great variety of toys and play-things: trolleys to push and hold on to while learning to walk, blocks to build with, wooden animals to sit in and rock, and many soft toys. There were two teenage school-girls down on the floor with them, who came, matron said, every day on a voluntary rota basis to stimulate the babies by play, to push them on the indoor or garden swings, to roll balls with them, shovel sand with them, splash water with them.

The youngest mongol was ten months old—a month younger than Lucy, but already sitting securely alone and playing with toys, obviously more advanced than Lucy. Strangely it comforted me to see another there less retarded than she. Somehow it helped me to feel justified in sending her there. A group of women from the local WI, matron told us, came in turn on fine mornings to take out in push-chairs and prams all those who were able to go out. It was one of the advantages, she said, of being in a middle-class residential area—the Lions Club were always willing to give practical help by putting things up in the garden or making things, and the Rotary Club would always raise money for anything they needed. I did not then realize what a rarity this was—what a small minority of institutions for the mentally handicapped received such help and support from the community; or indeed, what a rare person matron was to evoke such co-operation.

Matron told us herself the ratio of babies to staff—25 to 28—

and assured us that her nursing staff were fully qualified, and that a doctor called daily. We could see that here Lucy would have the best possible nursing and medical care, and as much as one could wish of play and stimulation and training. Would she need more? Affection perhaps? Matron told us that most of the nurses were resident and single, and gave the children more than physical care. 'They all', she said, 'have their own favourites and pets, to whom they give kisses and cuddles and play beyond the ordinary duty of a nurse.' It seemed an ideal place—and we realized that we were unusually lucky to have been offered it—but we could not rejoice.

Nothing to do then but wait. It was all settled. But was it? I could change my mind of course if I wanted to—I could tell them all that I did not want a place anymore, that I would keep Lucy at home. But did I want that? Was that the best for her and for us all? I went over and over in my mind the possible outcomes of either course and changed my mind daily. I consulted my conscience and examined my reasons, my motives, my responsibility. I doubted myself, my experience, my judgement, my instinct and my decisions.

Martin was very patient. He spoke to me reassuringly, reiterating our reasons and confirming the long-term wisdom of our decision—but after a time I began to notice him almost wince when I came back to the subject yet again, and he shied away from further discussion. Poor Martin. He, I knew, was not feeling so unshakably confident as he pretended. But we had chosen a path, and having chosen, Martin was prepared to follow it—while I strove unceasingly to discover the direction it took further and further ahead. I reminded myself of my favourite text, one which I remember from my earliest Sunday-school days and which I have had many occasions to recall—'There is always light enough to take the next step'. And this was the next step—so we must take it.

Certainly the change in her life would not disturb Lucy. There was no question that she knew me. Her little round wandering eyes rarely focused on anything for long. There was no sign at all that she distinguished people from things. She slept soundly all night and a great deal of the day—though asleep or awake it made little difference. Either way she lay quiet and inert, rarely crying, making no demands and no response. Frequently I took her out of her carry-cot to prop her in an armchair or lay her on the floor, but she hardly appeared to notice.

Now that Lucy had been offered a place and might be going quite soon, I wondered why I had been in such a hurry about it. If only I had known, could have been sure, that a suitable place was available to her, I could have kept her at home for a few years yet. But how would she or I react to it if or when she did know me? No, it was better this way.

And so for a short space longer I loved and cared for her, until a day came when Miss Fraser called again to say that a place was ready for Lucy—she was to go at the end of the week. So soon? I was devoured again by the doubt and emotional turmoil which was my usual reaction to anything concerning Lucy.

It was some time, therefore, before I noticed Julia's strange behaviour. She lay back in an armchair in a very awkward position staring straight ahead and looking very strained. She had been present when Miss Fraser told me the news, since we had only one living-room and anyway, she was too nervous to leave me. She had remained very quiet while Miss Fraser was there and had said nothing since. I spoke to her and she responded by asking when Daddy would be home. She retired even further into her chair, sucking her thumb in a way I had not seen her do for a very long time. I tried to interest her in something, but she said she just wanted to wait for Daddy, so I put on Andy Pandy while I fed and changed Lucy and prepared supper. When Martin came home she clung to him and said she was tired and wanted to go to bed. He was even longer than usual putting her to bed, and when he came down he said she seemed rather hot and he thought she was not very well. But she had run up casual temperatures so many times before that I was not over-concerned by this particular one, though in the further corners of my mind, where a little thought on things other than Lucy still went on, I was becoming perturbed by the whole pattern of them. Did not most of Julia's temperatures come on the days when Miss Fraser had been? or when I had been particularly upset? I could not remember exactly, and now I could wait no longer to tell Martin about Lucy going to Beechwood, and we could think of nothing else for the rest of the evening.

It was very obvious, next morning, that something was very wrong with Julia. Her cheeks were flushed and her eyes over-bright, her skin hot and dry. Again she was lying in a stiff awkward position, her left arm held tightly into her body and her head turned to the left. Martin spoke gently and soothingly to her and tried to move her, but she protested that she could not move. Alarmed, I fetched the thermometer and Martin took her temperature; with a sickening fear I saw that it was creeping towards the 105 mark. We phoned the doctor right away. She did not move all the morning but lay still and quiet and uncomplaining till the doctor arrived. He examined her gently and very thoroughly but was obviously puzzled. He could find no sign to explain her immobility. He took her temperature himself and then said that she must go into hospital right away. Fearful I asked him what he suspected, and he said, meditatively after a slight pause, that he thought it might be appendicitis. I was incredulous. She was reluctant or unable to move, and she had a very high temperature, but did that add up to appendicitis! He insisted that it could do, and that she may need an immediate operation.

I was convinced that there was nothing organically wrong with Julia. After all, she had quite often run up temperatures for no discernible reason, and had quickly recovered from them. I tried to tell Dr Baker about this but he was not interested. 'If it were my own daughter', he said, 'I should send her straight away.' I could not bear to let her go, and could not believe that it was necessary. I asked if we could have a second opinion, to which he replied that she would get that in hospital. When he spoke of laboratory tests I said we could take her to the hospital for tests and bring her home again—but he was adamant. At last

I agreed that we would take her, not because I had any intention of doing so, but because I could see that he would persist, and I could not bear any more pressure.

When he had gone I turned to Martin. 'You can't believe it,' I said, 'she can't possibly have appendicitis. We have seen her like this before—the only difference between now and those earlier occasions is one of degree, that's all; she has no other symptoms.' I was trying to rationalize something I felt in my bones—instinct or intuition—call it what you like, but I was convinced. Martin however, was not. He said that we had no alternative but to get her to hospital. Since Dr Baker had said that she may need an operation, we could not do otherwise: we could not stake her life on my instinct. Of course he was right. I gave in, and hurriedly we packed Lucy in her carry-cot, wrapped Julia in a blanket, and set off.

At the great ugly barrack-like building we were expected, and sister coldly showed us to a bed and told us to leave Julia quickly. We asked about visiting times and were handed a card stating that visiting was for half an hour daily, at seven o'clock in the evening. She told us firmly that visitors were not allowed on the ward at any other time. We asked to see the doctor, but were told that there was little point in that until the doctor had seen Julia—we could phone later. I gave Julia a hug as I tucked her into bed in the vast white ward—a strange environment to her—and she clung to my neck and cried, 'Mummy, Mummy, Mummy, don't leave me'. Sister was over instantly, insisting that we go, and pulling Julia's arms away from me. What could I do? I left quickly so as not to prolong the scene.

Nothing will ever erase from my mind the anguish I felt that day at leaving Julia in such a hostile environment. She was ill and she was desperately frightened. She needed me and Martin and the security of her own home, and all this was deliberately dragged from her. Was it really necessary to frighten her so much? Why could I not stay with her? When we arrived back at the car I was surprised to see Lucy there. I had quite forgotten about her. But she had not stirred—her eyes were open but she was not even aware that she had been left. I thanked God for her oblivion, and prayed that she would ever be so. She would never know the terror that Julia was facing now—never suffer the fears, the torments, the loneliness, the many hurts of life that must already be lying in wait for the sensitive highly-strung Julia.

How did we get through that day till visiting time? I cannot remember now. I can only remember that I was tormented. We phoned the hospital several times but got little information. At last we found ourselves with an anxious knot of parents crowded outside the door to the ward, waiting. I began to wonder what we were waiting for—it was so nearly seven o'clock. And at last a bell rang, and a starched nurse opened the doors, and viewed us suspiciously as we passed. 'Remember now,' she remonstrated, 'no sweets or food of any kind to be given to the children. No more than two at a time, and the bell will go at precisely seven-thirty.'

Julia was not in the bed where we had left her, and frantically we searched the long line of white strained children's faces. At last we picked her out and approached the bed, and talked to her and held out our arms. But she stared at us blankly, unknowing, much as Lucy did. Recognition came back after a little while, though it seemed like an eternity to me, and then she cried and clung to us, but feebly, distraught and despairing. She did not even ask to come home, as if she knew that was hopeless—or had she forgotten home already too? I put my arms around to cuddle her as she lay in bed, but sister passed by and looked at me sternly, so guiltily I released her. The bell rang and we had to tear ourselves away from her as she wept.

We went to the office and waited to see the doctor in a state of anguish. 'No,' he said when he came, seeming surprised at our question. 'No, there is no possibility that she has appendicitis, I think we can rule that out. We think she may have tonsillitis.' We were slightly astonished at the variance in diagnosis, but too worried to question it. 'If she does not need an operation couldn't she come home?' Martin asked. At this he looked thoughtful and said that in his opinion Julia could be looked after at home, but Dr Baker, knowing the family circumstances, had disagreed. We pressed him for an explanation, and he said that he understood that there was a mongol baby at home, and since these were highly susceptible to infection, Dr Baker could not agree to Julia coming home for fear that an undiagnosed infection might affect Lucy. We pointed out that Lucy would be going away in a few days, we told him of Julia's previous temperatures, of what care we would take to keep them apart— but he could only say that, since Dr Baker had refused to take over the care of Julia at home, he was unable to discharge her. There were, he said, various tests of her blood and urine under way, and he might have some better idea of what was wrong with her by tomorrow.

How did we get through that night, and the next day, and the next? For it went on and on. The doctor in charge of the ward, whom we had seen that first evening, himself went down with 'flu, and the ward depended entirely on young housemen, who had a host of different possible explanations of Julia's symptoms, and a host of different ways to test their hypotheses. Every day I made up my mind that we would simply bring Julia home with us, but every day there was one more horrible disease that they were testing for, so we had to leave her. Whenever we saw her she seemed more strange and distraught. The worst times were when she did not even cry, but just stared at us. A kindly coloured nurse told us that she cried and called for us all day long, and another confided that her temperature was falling but that her pulse was very rapid, and strongly advised us against removing her.

The day came to take Lucy to Beechwood. Apathetically we packed her belongings, and set off to drive through the rain. We took her in, in her carry-cot, and matron showed us to the room which she was to share. I tucked her in, and tucked in too the few soft toys I had brought. I put in Lucy's hand the piece of soft cloth she liked to hold—it was the nearest she had come to using a plaything. I explained to matron her feeding habits and all the little details of her care. We kissed her goodbye—but she did not know it—she gave no sign at all that she was aware of her changed environment. We left then and I cried softly as I walked back through the house, not even caring if anyone saw me. And then matron came hurrying after us with the maroon carry-cot that Lucy had almost lived in for so long. 'You'd better take this,' she said brightly, 'she won't be needing it now.' And with that I broke down and wept uncontrollably. It seemed to me the cruellest blow, to deprive little Lucy of her cot. Silly of course, but it brought home to me the change that was coming into her life, and the fact that I was no longer able to control the details of it.

And so we went home alone, with the empty cot, and waited for the hours to pass until we could visit Julia.

Chapter 9

IN ALL MY life I have never suffered so acutely as I did that next week. Not in the many months I have spent in hospital myself, not in the times when I have been lonely, or frightened, or distressed about my loved ones; nothing was or could ever be more devastating than having both the children taken from me. I remember when I was first ill myself, in my teens, just after my father died. In a critical condition I was sent to a large sanatorium, a hostile environment where the teenage factory girls I was with delighted in mocking me for my seriousness. That was a hell I felt I could not endure. It was about the time of the Nuremberg trials, when the newspapers were full of the horrifying details of the concentration camps. I wondered how people had borne it. How could any endure? Surely I never could. I persuaded myself that each of us must have a certain capacity for suffering limited by a threshold that could not be crossed whatever happened to us; a threshold beyond which one became insensitive, anaesthetized, to pain or suffering. And I felt then that my threshold was nearly reached—that if I went from my National Health sanatorium to a concentration camp, I could not suffer very much more. That must be the explanation I thought, or at least, I hoped. But I had not then had the experience of having one's young children in hospital, not knowing if they would ever come home again. Martin felt as deeply as I, though he bore it more stoically.

Somehow the time passed. Martin occupied himself making Julia a doll's house, calmly and deftly working to his own meticulous standard of craftsmanship. I was shocked when he reminded me that it would soon be Christmas. Another Christmas? Would Julia be home in time for Christmas? or would she be dead by then? Or—an even more terrifying thought—was she suffering some dreaded disease that would leave her crippled or imbeciled for life? On one occasion we went to the town and while Martin was buying his wood for the doll's house, I went across to the baker's. I stood on the pavement waiting to cross the busy main road, and then suddenly found myself stepping out in front of an oncoming car. I fell, quite involuntarily I think, and lay there in its path—but there was only a screech of brakes, a passer-by picking me up, and an excited driver shouting at me. I hobbled back to the car, both my knees badly bruised and waited for Martin, almost regretting that the accident had not taken me out of life's arena altogether.

At last there came a time when the doctors said Julia could come home. Her temperature was still raised in spite of the quantities of antibiotics they had pumped into her; and in spite of the multiplicity of tests they made, they could find no evidence of illness. The young housemen had wanted to keep her till her temperature fell, but when the paediatrician returned he concluded that her temperature was unlikely to fall while she was so distressed, so she should come home.

It was a strange child we fetched home. Pale and solemn, silent and unresponsive, she sat like a little wax doll. I sat on the back seat with her and tried to cuddle her, but she was stiff and unbending. At home we tried to cheer her by getting down her dolls and toys. Since her temperature was still high we had been told to keep her in bed, but instead we got cushions and rugs and lay her on the sofa so that we could both be with her, and she could see all that was going on. Martin tried to get some response from her; he called her Pampadouzle, his old pet name for her, and got out the wooden ark he had made for her previously, making up stories about the animals as he walked them up the ramp. But Julia did not smile or take any part.

I prepared her favourite lunch, an old family dish we called Saxon Stew, rabbit and lentils and dumplings, but she only became petulant when it was offered, so we did not press her to eat. We hoped she would sleep in the afternoon but she stayed wide-eyed. It was not till the dark had fallen, and we had drawn the curtains, and turned the glowing coals, and were making toast for tea, that the frozen personality cracked—then she sat up on the sofa and began banging her head repeatedly on the hard sofa-back. Concerned we rushed to her, and Martin scooped her up in his arms and held her tight while she struggled. And then as he nursed her she cried, a long quiet hopeless sobbing which did not stop till she had fallen asleep, her white face puffy with crying, and her curls wet with her tears. We realized then, that young and small as she was, she had known real suffering in the past two weeks. Limited in knowledge and understanding a young child may be, but capable of suffering—perhaps as much as ever in later years.

Julia's strange withdrawn behaviour persisted unchanged for days, and then began to recede only slowly over the succeeding weeks and months and years. For the next week or so she continued to bang her head against the sofa, the walls, the head of her bed, whenever she was distressed, and she would jump up screaming and run to the farthest corner of the house whenever she heard a car in the courtyard, thinking it was a doctor come to send her to hospital. Her fear at the sound of cars in the court-yard persisted for several years, and her extreme fear of doctors has lasted through all her childhood. It is only now, as she goes into her teens, that she is beginning to be able to accept them rationally.

We had intended to tell Julia about Lucy's going away, and to explain it to her in a way we hoped she would be able to under stand. But Julia's behaviour was so strange that it did not seem wise. She herself did not mention, or even seem to notice, that Lucy was no longer there. We had not wanted Lucy to go while Julia was away, so that she came home from hospital to find that Lucy had just disappeared. It would, we thought, have been better to delay Lucy's going, so that sometime after Julia's return we could all take her together. Julia had always been so protective towards Lucy that it would not be easy for her to accept the idea of Lucy going away, but we hoped that seeing Lucy settled unprotestingly in such a nice place, Julia would at least have seen that Lucy was happy and well-cared-for. But Dr Baker's concern about infection had made that impossible. And so it was a fortnight or so before we dared to speak to Julia about Lucy, and when we did tell her she received the news without comment; no questions, no 'whys', no demands to go to see her —none of the battery of comment she would most certainly have subjected us to before she had been in hospital.

We had been given an appointment to take Julia to the out-patients' department a fortnight after her discharge, and once again Martin and I disagreed about what to do. It was rare for us to differ; usually we could act happily in concert. It seemed glaringly obvious to me now that Julia had been seriously disturbed and distressed in hospital, that she had had no real illness, that in fact her temperature and immobility were hysterical reactions to the stress she was under from my own tension and behaviour, from the aura of anxiety that surrounded Lucy on our frequent visits to the doctor, and finally, from the fear she must have felt when she heard Miss Fraser speak of Lucy going away.

It was to be expected that a visit to the out-patients' department would cause her further distress, and, as far as I could see, to no purpose. Martin, however, was still anxious lest there were some physical disease not yet diagnosed. He could not believe that a child could be so very ill simply from fear or anxiety. Certainly, I had been very slow to recognize it myself, in spite of my professional training. But I knew now, as I had feared all along, that Julia was being deleteriously affected by our emotional upheaval over Lucy, and by my exclusive involvement with her. For Julia this last experience of being separated from us in such a way had been traumatic. If psychologists were right about the life-long influence of our experiences in early years, then the damage might be irreparable.

In spite of Martin's extreme protectiveness towards Julia, and his reluctance to cause her more distress, he was so worried about the possibility of serious physical disease, that he insisted that we go. And so we wrapped her up in a blanket and took her in the car. We dared not tell her where we were going, which was quite against our usual practice of explaining everything to her at a level she would understand. But we knew there was no level at which she could understand or accept this.

As soon as the car drew up outside the hospital she recognized where she was, and screamed to Martin, 'Daddy, go on, go on, Daddy, don't stop, no, no, no'. We held her tight while she struggled to make Martin drive on, and then Martin held her to get her out of the car, but she clung desperately with all her strength to the seats, the door, to me. Six-feet-two and broad and strong, Martin had difficulty in holding her. But he carried her in, and we sat and waited in the hot waiting-room, Julia still clutching the rug around her and over her head. At last we went in to see the paediatrician. Seeing the rug he asked if she were still ill, but we explained that she was holding it there for protection, and understanding, he did not come near or disturb her. The young houseman with him began talking about urine-test results which he said were 'equivocal', but the paediatrician cut him short to question us about Lucy—her going to Beechwood, and the circumstances leading up to Julia's illness. 'I don't think there is any doubt,' he said, 'that Julia's illness is psychosomatic. You must do what you can to reassure her. Give her all the attention you can. Keep her quietly at home for the next two or three months to enable her to recover, then take her along to the Child Guidance Clinic. I think you were wise,' he went on, 'to get Lucy away, but you kept her too long, didn't you?'

We tried then to settle down into our old family life again, but we were no longer the same people. We took the paediatrician's advice and did what we could to rehabilitate Julia. As the weeks went by her personality slowly thawed, but she had regressed a great deal. She reverted to many babyish ways, sucking her thumb, toying with her food, wetting the bed, and now we actually had to stimulate her to take an interest in things, whereas previously, since her very birth, she had been the one to stimulate us.

Earlier she had made precocious development. By her second birthday she had recited the whole of a Ladybird story book, turning the correct pages as she went, appearing to read it. At the place where we waited for Daddy to come off-duty, she quickly learned to recognize the words of the notice, 'Do not proceed beyond this point,' and from that she had started to read almost spontaneously. She had joined the public library and spent a long time there with Martin choosing new books which he read to her at bed-time; but now, at three and three-quarters, she reverted to listening passively to the same stories she had listened to half her life-time ago.

It was a passive period for me too. With Lucy away I hardly thought about her. Indeed I deliberately shut out all thought of her—and left Martin to phone for news. The extreme sense of guilt I had felt was refuelled now by the feeling that I had rejected Lucy, and by the knowledge of what my emotional reaction to Lucy had done to Julia.

But as time went by we both began to recover. I started to take Julia down into the village to a combined coffee-morning play-group, where she and I could both meet others, and although she clung to me instead of playing with the other children, and I felt awkward and estranged from their mothers, it did bring us back into society.

Martin began to take her with him to the library again, and he always looked out for a well-illustrated book to show her— birds, fishing, travel, history, he found interesting pictures on every conceivable subject. He interested her in other activities too. When he decided to paint the outside of the house white, he let Julia have a go first. With a large house-painting brush and old clothes that would not be needed again, he encouraged her to slosh the paint over the walls in arm-length sweeps— and she did. She enjoyed it so much that we decided to give her the whole of the white-painted kitchen-door as a canvas, and Martin made her a little flight of steps so that she could reach to the top. We discovered that her own poster-paints easily washed off the high-gloss surface, and it took her a long time to fill the space of the whole door with colour and pictures. For the effort of an occasional wash down, she was kept busy and happy in the kitchen for many hours while I was cooking or washing-up.

The time came when Martin remarked that we really ought

to go to see Lucy. I did not want to see her; I did not want to think about her. I wanted to forget her existence. Martin suggested that he went alone, and I was very tempted to let him, but I knew I had to go. So we went together one rainy afternoon, and had a painful scene when we tried to leave Julia. We were both of us consumed with anxiety about Lucy, although matron had told us on the phone that she was quite well.

She was lying on the floor on her tummy, and a nurse rushed over to move her, proudly demonstrating how she could nearly sit alone. Just as always her eyes wandered over us and away, but now she actually reached out for a bright toy near by—one we had bought for her first birthday. Certainly she seemed contented and well and making progress—but wasn't she a little thinner? I mentioned it to matron, and she said that, since Lucy was taking such vast quantities of milk, they thought she was ready for solid food, and were trying to introduce baby-cereals instead of some of the milk. Lucy however, was resisting this, and consequently was getting a reduced diet. Matron assured us that it was often a problem getting mongols to accept solid food, but she was sure Lucy would learn to take it soon. No harm would come to her, she assured us, Lucy could afford to lose a little fat. My heart sank at what seemed to me to be a harsh attitude, and it reminded me again that I had given over Lucy's care to others. I wept on the way home, and was distressed for many days.

By our second visit Lucy was looking plumper and pinker, since they had abandoned their efforts to make her take solid food and reverted to an all milk diet. She was sitting steadily now, on the floor with the other children, and suddenly looking more like them—a toddler rather than a baby. She was contented, well, and making progress, but it was nevertheless a most painful experience. We continued to make painful erratic visits, always preceded by days of anxiety, and followed by days of depression. I could quite understand why so many mentally-handicapped children were placed in homes and then abandoned by their families—why their families moved away without trace. It was not because they did not care—but because they cared too much. It would be so much easier to cut a child out of one's life altogether than to reopen the wound at every visit.

Soon our relatives and friends got to know that Lucy was away, and they all expressed their views on it. Almost invariably the men were warm and convincing in assuring us that we had done the right thing—and we craved for approval—but from the women the reaction was different. None dared to tell us we were wrong—an accusation against which we could have defended ourselves—but several said what seemed to me worse, 'Oh I'm sure', they said, 'that you are absolutely right. It's just that I could not have done it.' And I felt more alien than ever.

On a sunny day in early spring we set off to take Julia to the woods—and found the courage to call and collect Lucy too. Julia was quiet when we first showed her where Lucy was, and thoughtful when she saw Lucy in the car with us again. She was bigger and sturdier now, her head held erect, and she was outgrowing the yellow sleeping-bag I had made for her. She gazed round the car and looked at us in an interested way, and responded with a gurgle and a smile when Julia played with her. In the woods she studied the twigs as we passed, and watched Julia and Martin gathering the first catkins. We went to a country inn for tea, always a special delight for Julia, and Lucy was able to sit up on my lap instead of lying inert in her carry-cot.

It was a very successful afternoon. For the first time I felt almost happy as I left Lucy. There did, after all, seem to be a way that she could live a separate sheltered life away from us, and yet remain a part of the family.

But after we were home, Julia was still thoughtful. 'Why can't Lucy come home, Mummy? I wish she could.' And the next day she ran up a high temperature again, and she was cranky and disturbed for two more.

We felt it was important to maintain a close family link with Lucy, and hoped that in time Julia would be able to accept the situation without fretting. So we made a habit of taking Lucy out with us whenever we could.

Matron was always happy to let her come at a moment's notice, and we were reassured by this that Lucy was as well cared for when we were not there as when we went on our arranged visits. Julia continued to question us about Lucy, and we tried to explain it to her in a way that she would understand. We told her it was better for Lucy to be with others like herself, and to have the nurses to look after her. 'But what is it,' Julia insisted, 'that the nurses can do for Lucy that we can't?' I was hard-pressed to answer that one—nevertheless she did seem to accept the situation.

In May Julia was four, and by then she seemed so much improved that I delayed going to the Child Guidance Clinic. There was no possibility, yet, of getting her back to the play-group, as she still would not leave me, but I was finding more opportunities for her to meet other children, and now that Martin and I were more relaxed, she was slowly regaining something of her old personality.

She was an imaginative child. I remember a day that summer when we walked in the hay-field, the pollen from the grass blowing in white clouds about us as we walked. Julia imagined she had found a rabbit. 'Save a bit of apple for my rabbit,' she told me, 'tell him we have not brought a gun.' She made up a story about him, babbling on as we walked in the sun, the bees droning around us. I was thinking of other things, my mind tuning in and out to Julia, catching only snatches of the story— '. . . so he packed his suitcase of woven grass with his clothes made of buttercups and clover . . .' She saw a brown and black butterfly and tried to remember its markings so that Daddy could look it up in the book.

She was a serious child too. 'I think till my ears are full of thinks,' she told me, and there were many days when she was low-spirited: 'Oh Mummy,' she would say to me then, 'I feel so sad today. I just want to crawl back inside your tummy and go to sleep.'

Out in the copse we came across a dead pigeon which aroused Julia's curiosity. 'How do you know, Mummy, that it is dead and not just sleeping? What is the difference, Mummy, between being asleep and being dead? Will Daddy die, Mummy? Will you? Will I really be quite grown up, Mummy, before you and

Daddy die?' They were all just questions provoked by her
curiosity, I thought, and by a very natural fear of being left
alone, but the same subject cropped up again and again in a
variety of situations. 'Julia, Julia,' I called one evening after she
had been playing in the bath for an unusually long time, 'come
along. It's time you were out.' 'You count up to the number of
years a person lives till he dies,' she said, 'and then I'll get out
of the bath.' Did all four-year-olds talk like this, I wondered?
Were they all so obsessed by the idea of death?

Although she was so much more stable in behaviour than she
had been around the time of her illness, yet I was vaguely
worried. I had little confidence by then in my ability and instinct
as a mother, so at last I took the paediatrician's advice and went
to the Child Guidance Clinic.

I was very glad that I did. It was one of the most worthwhile
things I did at that time. Whether or not it made much difference to Julia I am not sure, but it did a great deal for me.

I went alone at first, and saw an ageing psychiatric social
worker, Miss Beamish, a lady of great experience, insight and
sensitivity. She had already had a report about Julia from the
hospital, and suggested that I bring her regularly every week
to see the child-psychologist upstairs in the play-room. I was to
stay with Julia until she was confident enough to stay without
me, then I should come downstairs and talk to Miss Beamish.

Our first conversation was a bit stilted. I felt rather resentful
when she asked me about my own childhood, yet quickly found
that I was telling her all about Melanie. By the second meeting
I was telling her unreservedly all I felt about Lucy, and of how I
had wanted and even tried to kill her.

What a blessed relief it was to confess that. And to find that
one had done it without causing so much as a raised eyebrow
from the imperturbable Miss Beamish. What a balm is confession! Suddenly I understood a lot more about the Roman
Catholic Church. Confession itself is a therapy. Yet I felt no
guilt about my viewpoint, only the need to confess to an opinion
for which most of society would condemn me.

We continued to attend the clinic for some time—Julia happily playing upstairs while I talked to Miss Beamish. At the end of it I was myself feeling a great deal more confident, more positively me, more secure in my right to hold the opinion I did; and I was beginning to come to terms with the practical compromise with society that I had made in sending Lucy away. Julia too, was beginning to blossom again, though whether this was the direct result of her sessions with the psychologist and play-therapist, or the effect of my own improved state I do not know. Either way, all credit to the clinic.

Miss Beamish helped me to face the conflict of loyalty I felt towards the children. She reminded me that it was Julia's needs which were paramount then. 'Lucy,' she said, 'will never be so sensitive or so vulnerable as Julia is now. Lucy's needs at this stage are simple, mainly physical, and they are being adequately met at Beechwood. Julia on the other hand, is already showing signs of emotional insecurity which, if it continues, might affect her for the rest of her life. No-one but you can help Julia.'

Julia was obviously, she said, a highly intelligent child, well in advance of most children of her age, but she was also a highly sensitive one, with many qualities of character already apparent which would make her a uniquely valuable member of society if she was not warped by fear and unhappiness now. Children of Gold, she said Plato called them, and society neglects them at its peril.

I tried to put my guilt from me, and accept Julia as my first priority. Life, I realized, was not something that was going to happen to Julia tomorrow. Life was now.

Chapter 10

WHEN SUMMER WAS high and the chestnut blossom petals thick upon the lawn, we met Alice and Wendy. I was pushing Julia on the swings one day, in the gardens in the middle of the town, and Alice was doing the same for her daughter Wendy. Wendy was about Julia's age, shy and quiet, and Alice was concerned that Wendy had no play-mates since the family had only recently come to the town where they knew no-one.

Alice immediately invited us back to their rented flat, and asked if I knew of a house which they were then in the throes of buying. 'Is that,' she said, 'anywhere near the area where you live?' It was—very near—separated only by a field and a wood on a hill; muddy most of the year but certainly accessible. We became firm friends, Alice and I, and Julia and Wendy, and from that day on saw each other regularly for the next five years until they left the district.

Wendy spent a lot of time at our house that summer—it was so convenient for Alice to leave Wendy with us while she went to clean and measure and prepare their new house.

I put up the red wigwam which Joanne had sent for Julia's birthday, and Martin made a tripod of logs for a fire over which they hung cooking-pots full of weeds and stones. They took a wide variety of dolls and animals and utensils in with them and played in the most imaginative way. It was the sort of play which involved them totally for many hours, and obviously needed intense concentration—they were as impatient of interruption as any business executive. Often I left them with bottles of squash and packets of sandwiches to avoid disturbing them for meals.

The two children became inseparable. For the next few years they clung to each other, almost exclusive of other friends. Later on they began to spend odd nights in each other's homes, and liked to pretend that they were sisters.

Alice and I became good friends too, although we were so different, and one might have thought we had little in common. She was a happy outgoing vivacious person, who had many interests and pursued them energetically. She was an attractive and sociable person, and soon knew far more people in the village than I ever did. She took life lightly, while I was so intense, yet we did become friends, and her friendship meant a great deal to me in the next years.

Their house was high on a steep south-facing hill overlooking the valley and the village, and was surrounded by woodland. It was approached by an unmade road which needed a good pair of lungs or a powerful engine to ascend it, but was worth the effort if one liked seclusion, beautiful scenery, and a rural life. Alice and Bob, her husband, were keen gardeners, as had been their predecessors, and soon Wendy and Julia were up there helping to pick the beans and the raspberries.

Alice and I took the children out often, to the beach, to the park, to gymkhanas and village fêtes. The fête in our own village we would not miss. It had been held for centuries on the same green, bringing all the villagers together for the same sort of festivity. Changes had been slight and had crept in only slowly over the decades. There was the same maypole dancing by the village children, the same display of flowers and vegetables, of cakes and preserves, of eggs and honey; and then there was the same tug-of-war between men from different sides of the river, and the same bowling for a pig—except that now one had the option, should one be skilful enough to win it, of taking a cash payment instead of the pig.

Under Martin's guidance Julia and Wendy were busy for several days before collecting their grasses to enter in the 'Collection and Arrangement of Grasses' competition, and making their miniature gardens in soup plates. They collected 29 different grasses each, and one of them took a third prize, and the other a prize for her miniature garden. They joined in the races too, sack and potato, and watched the Punch and Judy show, and had a pony ride, and sucked ice-lollies while the farmers' lads competed at pitching the hay.

In early September we had Lucy home to stay for a few days. What joy it was then to have her at home; and what a basic satisfaction there was in tending her. Relieved of the worry about her future, or the hope of her death, caring for her was a very different experience. She smiled and gurgled in her bath, and slooped lustily on her bottle, and obviously enjoyed watching Julia and Wendy as she sat on a rug in the garden. We sat her near the wigwam and they included her in their play—though that of course meant nothing to Lucy, except that she noticed their coming and going. Obviously, we assured ourselves, she was well and happy, and progressing quite as well at Beechwood as she was likely to have done at home.

We were encouraged by Lucy's progress at Beechwood and began to feel that we had been justified in sending her there; the secret shame we had both felt about it began to fade. Thus emboldened, and feeling I wanted to be involved in anything relating to the mentally handicapped, I went again to the Mencaps—that is, my local branch of the Society for the Mentally Handicapped.

It was over a year since my earlier visits, but still a few people recognized and spoke to me. During coffee they asked about Lucy—and I told them she was away. Instantly there was silence—cold voices and set faces. No one asked about her further. No one asked where, or when, or why. The subject was closed and they turned to talk among themselves, leaving me feeling slightly baffled and distinctly snubbed.

I retired from the group, since I was obviously not included in their conversation, and an elderly well-spoken lady came over to me. As if in apology for the group she said that they met infrequently and had a lot of news to catch up on. 'Everyone wants to talk to Mrs Coleman,' she said,' to enquire about her son.' And she told me about him.

Mrs Coleman had a son, Peter, aged sixteen, a brilliant boy who had won a scholarship to the direct-grant grammar school. She also had at home a mentally-handicapped daughter of about twelve, Pam, of whom Peter was very fond. For some time the boy had been behaving very strangely—not making friends at school, not having any interests outside the home. He had taken to playing truant from school, and his masters were puzzled about such behaviour from an obviously able boy. It had culminated in his taking an overdose of his mother's sleeping pills in a suicide attempt. He was taken to hospital where they pumped out his stomach, and after a little time at home, unable to face school-life, he had been admitted to a mental-hospital where he was having electrical treatment. His sister Pam, at home without him, was pining; he had used to spend so much time with her.

It was a sad story. I felt deeply sorry for Mrs Coleman. Of course, I did not know enough of the facts to make a judgement, but I could not help suspecting that the presence of his handicapped sister was at least a contributory factor in his inability to relate to his peers, if not the whole of it. It reminded me so much of the way I had, at that age, isolated myself from society to be with Melanie.

By the end of the evening, when the group who had been so cold to me were melting a little and I was included again, it was Mrs Coleman herself who gave me a clue to the reason why they had shunned me. 'I have been shouldering my burden,' she said, 'for twelve long years. Every day, week after week, month after month, year after year, I have had to bear my cross myself. You have got rid of yours.' So even here I was an outcast.

At Christmas Lucy came home again to spend the holiday and her second birthday with us. She was plump and contented as usual, much as she was in September.

On Boxing Day we all went to see the hunt meet, Lucy well snuggled up in Martin's arms. It was a colourful spectacle and we were stimulated by the frosty air and the excitement of the hounds. We followed for a while and saw the fox speed across a field and take cover in a wood. The hounds who had been on the scent, soon lost it.

After Christmas it began to snow, and Martin took Julia and Wendy out tobogganing. The hillside fields around our home were ideal for that, and people came to them from the town bringing sledges and skis. I was grateful for living in such a lovely country setting, in spite of the many times I had complained of the inconvenience of being so far from shops and services.

Julia and Wendy started taking dancing lessons together on Saturday mornings, Alice and I taking turns to accompany them. They danced with the same serious concentration that they did everything else, yet they enjoyed it immensely—it was impossible to persuade them to miss a morning when one of them had a cold, or the roads were icy.

In Spring Martin suggested that we rear some chicks. We bought three day-olds—pullets we hoped. We wanted the laying hens, but we also wanted the children to have the experience of seeing something develop from birth to maturity, and with hens you can see a lot of development in a short space of time. At first we had to have them in the house, with a light bulb under a flower-pot to keep them warm. They cheeped and pecked busily all day long, and seemed to work very hard at growing up. They delighted the children, who were forever round their box handling them and feeding them or just watching them.

When they had grown a bit and were fully feathered, we transferred them to part of the garden and Martin turned an old water-butt on its side for use as a coop. He hinged the lid to make a door and filled it up with fresh hay and we shut them up there at night. Julia and Wendy crawled in themselves sniffing the exotically scented hay, and declaring they would like to sleep there. The pullets grew rapidly until they were sleek and red and plump, and followed the girls round the garden as faithfully as any pet. But as soon as dusk threatened they would make their own way back to their barrel, and we only needed to go down and shut their door.

When they were about four months old the inevitable happened. There came a night when we forgot to go and shut

4

them in—and the fox came. In the morning we found one bedraggled and befuddled hen perched in a tree, and only scattered feathers to indicate the fate of the other two.

We were all so unhappy about it that we went back to the farm where we had bought them, and were able to get two more of exactly the same age as our own. Indeed, the farmer assured us, they came from the very same batch. But when we were shown the pen where they were we thought there must be some mistake. These were not so large and plump as ours—even their faces looked more pinched. But the farmer was convinced that they were the same batch, and he seemed surprised that we had reared all three in spite of the children handling them.

When we released our two new hens in the garden they seemed rather bewildered, and wandered aimlessly about, not pecking and scraping the ground and working hard at life as the others had done. Our one survivor was certainly changed; she rarely came down from her perch and remained aloof from the others. We thought at first it was the strangeness of the new situation for them all, which made their behaviour so different, and that with time that would change. But it did not. I had never before thought much about animal personality, and if pressed would probably have said that a hen did not have one, but the dramatic change in our survivor indicated what a traumatic experience she had undergone. The night with the fox and the separation from her companions changed her behaviour altogether, and although we kept them for two years, she never recovered her old personality.

The two newcomers grew fatter and started laying, but they stayed always together and shunned the survivor, and never themselves became the real pets that the lost ones had been. What an interesting study that would be, I thought, for a student of personality and relationships.

Julia started school in the week that she was five. Unfortunately Wendy, a few months younger, was not to start till a term later. We chose a small fee-paying convent school, after a great deal of enquiry and heart-searching, because the classes were much smaller and it seemed a gentler environment.

Education came very high on our list of priorities—it was something we would willingly have given up cars or dogs or holidays for—so we had visited all the schools in our area, state and private, and chose the one we thought would suit Julia best.

Nevertheless, she did not fit into school easily. The playground frightened her, and she was over-anxious to please her teachers. Like many bright children she found school restrictive and tedious, and was overwhelmed by the assertiveness of children who herded together more instinctively than she did. She dutifully played with water and sand, and fitted shapes into boxes and painted, but in reading and writing and number work she was suddenly halted in her tracks—and made to fret and worry about adding one to one, when previously she had talked casually in thousands. 'You must not,' she told me when she was nearly six, and having difficulty in adding two to three, 'go faster than the teacher.' And so it was for the next year or so. School did little to stimulate or excite or enlarge her, only to instil in her a need to conform, which she was ill equipped to do.

But she adapted to it quite well. In fact, for almost the first time in her life she started to sleep right through the night. Until then we had grown accustomed to her being awake and playing from about two a.m. till four.

We continued to have Lucy home for a few days now and again, and to visit her frequently. She grew plump and bonny and continued to make slow progress. She began to smile a lot, and then to laugh infectiously and often. She was walking by about three and a bit, and soon progressed to running, though she could not manage stairs. She continued to need nappies, and had to wear bibs for a long time; her chin was always wet with dribbling.

The feeding problem recurred several times during those early years at Beechwood—the nurses making recurrent attempts to get her on to solid food. They did not really succeed until she was four, and then only a limited amount of mush which had to be fed to her on a spoon.

It was lovely to take her out in those years when we were all together, and she could run and laugh. We took her often to the woods, the beach and the park. She loved people—any people— and if not restrained would run up to anyone she saw and reach out her arms to be lifted up, or would explore their bags and their pockets like a town-park squirrel.

I never restrained her if I saw her approaching elderly people —they were usually kind and indulgent—nor if she approached teenagers, who were always willing to play with her; but if I saw her approaching parents with young children, I rushed to retrieve her, knowing from experience that they would treat her coldly, and hasten to take their own children away.

This reaction was almost invariable, and could not have been more pronounced if she had had smallpox. Indeed I began to suppose that the parents believed mongolism to be infectious, so hastily did they rush to protect their offspring. But their action was not prompted by reason—they were responding instinctively, impelled by an innate impulse written into their genes, as old as life itself. Or perhaps, like our ancient ancestors, they regarded her as a changeling. Certainly she could be very Puckish! She would often grasp and pinch and punch using all her strength, laughing hilariously all the time, quite unaware of the pain she was causing.

For a long time she did not seem to know pain herself. Sometimes she would fall or knock herself in a way which would surely have caused another child to cry, but Lucy seemed unaware of it. It was only later that she began to notice, and then one could count to ten between the fall and the slow crumpling of her face to cry—but when that cry did come, it was the most pathetic and forlorn cry in the world. Often she hurt Julia, who bravely refused to cry herself and rarely hit back; and often she manhandled the cat, who quickly learnt to keep out of her way; or deliberately threw things around, enjoying the breaking and smashing. She shouted a great deal too, as uninhibitedly as she rushed about and hit out—but when she learned to kiss, she was equally uninhibited about that, and quickly acquired the habit of kissing and embracing everyone she met.

She was such a happy and affectionate child, who could not love her? Many did. At Beechwood as she grew she quickly became a favourite of the nurses, the school-girls, the visiting WI ladies. Often her own particular nurse would take Lucy home with her on her day off, and even her parents grew to love Lucy.

In an environment where few of the members made any response, Lucy's mischief, and her dampness at both ends, were easily compensated for by her sunny personality. Happiness is infectious—and Lucy was happy.

Chapter 11

IT WAS IN the summer when Lucy was four and a half that we began to worry about the future again. Beechwood was intended for babies under five, and Lucy was approaching that. What was to become of her then?

She had made tremendous progress at Beechwood; it had been an unqualified success. All the evidence pointed to the fact that Lucy was as happy and as complete a person there as she could have been at home; that she had developed as much as could possibly have been hoped for. She was certainly satisfied with herself.

Her stay at Beechwood had been as fortunate for us as it had been for her, enabling us, as it did, to maintain close contact with her. But where was she to go after her fifth birthday? Could we find another home that would suit her as well as Beechwood?

There was no comparable home that we knew of, so we started enquiring early. Perhaps it would have been better if we had not.

We spoke to matron, but she knew nothing but that Lucy would probably be moved some time after she was five, and in all probability, she said, it will be to Haughton.

Haughton was the institution for 1,500 inmates which we had first heard about from Dr Baker. It was at the other end of the county, 60 miles away. We had heard a great deal more of it from the parents at the Mencap Society, who all knew of some past or present inmate, and who held the place in some abhorrence.

We became very alarmed then, and sought information from every possible source about other possibilities. There was another small place for children like Lucy, we discovered, Plumfield, in a small ancient town by the sea, perhaps 30 or 40 miles away. Hopefully I enquired about it at the Mencaps, whose meetings I still attended from time to time, but was confused by very conflicting reports they gave me.

I phoned Miss Fraser to ask her advice and she put us in touch with the local mental health officer. We spoke to him about Plumfield, and said that we would like to visit it to consider whether to apply for a place there. He was kindly, but offputting. He said that Plumfield was outside our area; that they were full; that they would undoubtedly have a waiting list of several years. We should, he said, consider ourselves lucky if Lucy were given a place at Haughton, since there were countless mentally-handicapped children and adults at home for years because they could not get a place. He had many patients on his list who were 20 or 30 years old, and whose ageing parents could hardly cope with them longer, but there was just nowhere to send them.

We pressed him for information of other homes, state or private, but there was none within 100 miles or so, and he knew of nothing beyond that.

He urged us to accept a place at Haughton if it were offered, and feel grateful for it. 'It is not so bad,' he said, 'as some people make out. Of course when you see so many of them together it's a bit of a shock at first, but they are quite happy and well-cared-for.' He told us that it was an estate covering many acres, with separate buildings for the different departments. The children's section, he said, was split into several cottages each containing 20 or 30 children, and from there they attended their own school-room. 'She'll be quite all right there,' he said, 'you have no need to worry.'

But we would not even consider that possibility. Determined to find some alternative, we wrote to the London Headquarters of the Mencaps to ask their advice. They sent us lists of other associations which might possibly be able to help, and a list of private homes, but they were not very hopeful. We wrote to every single one of the different associations on the list, but none of them could help. We wrote to a vast number of private homes, but these seemed to be under as great a pressure for places as the

National Health institutions. Only one or two, very far afield, had even the distant possibility of a vacancy, and the fees were staggeringly high. The average cost of the places at that time was considerably greater than the cost of keeping a boy at Eton. Only in the case of a Mencap child, of course, the expense would continue for life, not just for the handful of school years.

That was quite impossible for us, but since I had just started teaching again we could manage to pay a reasonable proportion, and appealed to the authorities for a grant to pay the balance. This, apparently, was quite out of the question. Either the local authority approved of sending your child to a private home, in which case it paid the total fees regardless of your own income; or it did not, in which case it paid nothing. In this case my local authority would not consider my, or any other, application, because it had Haughton.

There seemed nothing else to do but wait and hope that the authorities themselves would have an alternative when the time came.

The time came much earlier than we had expected. It was in September, when Lucy was just four and three-quarters, that a letter came simply stating that she would be transferred within a fortnight to Haughton. We phoned immediately to ask if we could visit Haughton and went within a day or two..

The first shock comes when, driving by a high brick wall for half a mile, you discover that it secures not violent criminals, but children like Lucy—together with those others who make up the one and a half thousand. Inside the gates and a long way up the drive one begins to see a few men ambling about. Men with unkempt hair, shirt necks flapping, flies undone, wearing carpet slippers and with self-rolled cigarettes hanging limply from their lips, either that or with mouths sagging open or perhaps dribbling. Leaving the men's section behind we began to see women looking equally repellent. Their dress was as slovenly as the men's, their figures either grossly fat and flabby or, skinny and wasted. All alike seemed to be slouching about in soft slippers, and all were wearing old-fashioned pinafores. Many were smoking or had dyed and matted hair. Occasionally they had some obvious physical deformity as well. But the most horrifying of all was the uniformity of their blank faces. Is this what my little Lucy would grow into?

We were shown around the various departments by someone who was introduced to us as a nurse, though she wore no precise uniform, only an anonymous white coat. She too had dyed blonde hair and a dangling cigarette, and apart from the white coat was hardly distinguishable from the patients.

After the sight of the people outside, it was almost a relief to get inside the buildings—at least there was a recognizable hospital atmosphere, though the smell was very strange and faintly nauseating. It was bare and bleak in the extreme, and we were shown only a few rooms which were unoccupied at the time.

Out on to the green again, and more women standing about, but this time they stared at us amiably as we passed, and one or two smiled and waved. We were told that these were the 'higher grade' patients who came to the children's blocks to help with the cleaning and feeding.

We went on to the block of school-rooms, and there the children showed signs of animation which were a welcome contrast to the apathetic wandering of the adults we had seen. They were happily occupied with paint and paste and the walls were bright with their own work. The teacher was young and alert, and we greeted her with some relief at meeting a recognizable fellow-being.

Our guide left us then, so we were free to talk to the teacher, Miss Hopkins, and her kindly assistants in the other classrooms. The numbers of children had outstripped the school's capacity, so some groups of children came in for only the mornings or afternoons. They came at any age when they could join in the activities, which were all the usual nursery school activities but with a stronger emphasis on practical skills like learning to dress themselves, tie laces, do up buttons, manage cutlery; and skills of an occupational value like sewing and knitting; and some things they did just for fun, like singing. They did quite a lot of speech work at the school too, as they were unable to get a

4*

speech-therapist, and a large proportion of the children spoke little or indistinctly.

There was a domestic science centre, we were told, for the older girls, but unfortunately that was closed at the moment because they were unable to get staff. Miss Hopkins was worried about the effect of the half-day, since for the other half the pupils remained unoccupied on the wards. But she was hopeful that something might be done to resolve the problem soon.

We were very impressed by the school, and by the obvious dedication of Miss Hopkins and her staff. Certainly, the very animation of the children was evidence of the school's positive value. When one was inside the school-rooms the whole prospect seemed quite different; bright, hopeful, optimistic.

One of the assistants took us to the occupational therapy block, and there too was a vigorous active environment. The patients were older, dishevelled and unattractive, but they were engrossed in the leather and cane ware they were creating. The therapist too, was a dedicated person, frantically busy and very concerned. She told us how involved her pupils were with their work, and how frustrating it was for them to be able to do it on only one day a week. I asked why this was and the answer was the same, too few facilities and too few staff to cope with the vast numbers. 'In the old days,' she said, 'many of these patients would have died in infancy, or would not have survived beyond their teens, but modern medical facilities are keeping them alive, and we cannot cope with the flood.' Many of the patients had no work or occupation of any kind for long periods of time. There were many 'difficult' patients who had behavioural problems, and these were always most pronounced among those with least to do.

We thanked the staff and left then, sated with our conflicting impressions. It needed, we both felt, a period of tranquillity away from it to allow the process of mental-digestion to take place.

We were quiet together on the long drive home. We stopped for tea, indulging ourselves a little after our emotional battering, but even then we did not talk about it.

It was in bed very early the next morning when I brought the subject up, and Martin was still muzzy with sleep. 'We can't possibly send her there,' I said, and he was instantly alerted. 'My dear,' he said, 'we must. Oh I know what you are thinking. I know what you feel. To you it was appalling—and to me. But those children we saw were happy. They do not see it with our eyes. They are not affronted as we are by the sight of those forgotten aimless people. To them the attention and concern of those dedicated teachers is a much more positive thing. The swings and see-saws in the garden, the older friendly patients who help them and are kind to them—these are the positive things that will matter to Lucy.

'You know, my dear, that we have no alternative, and we must try to judge it from her needs, not ours.'

Certainly it was true we had little alternative, there was in fact only one—to keep her at home. We had been over that possibility a thousand times. She was so boisterous and mischievous now that she needed constant attention. She could not be left unsupervised anywhere for even a few seconds, she was so unpredictable, so uninhibited, and so strong.

There was no hope that she could attend a Day Training Centre, now or ever, even though they were building one in the next town. It was already subscribed several times over, and Lucy, we were told, would not be eligible because of the degree of handicap.

At the back of our minds was the certain knowledge that, if we refused the place at Haughton now, and kept her at home, she was unlikely to be offered a place again until we were too senile to look after her longer.

'Think', said Martin, 'what that first year did to you and to Julia. Yes, and to me too. We cannot go through that again. It will eat away at all our lives like a cancer. No, she must go.

'And think of Lucy too,' he urged. 'She has done so well at Beechwood. She loves the company of the other children, she depends upon the strict routine—and as she gets older she will need some training, which at the Haughton school she will get. There will be nothing for her here but boredom, which she will relieve with her mischief. That's going to be a steadily growing problem as she gets bigger and stronger. It is for her benefit too, that she must go, not just ours.'

Again I suspected that Martin was trying as hard to convince himself as me, and I was sure of it when he suddenly said, 'Why don't we phone Miss Fraser, and ask if she could come down and talk it over with us. I think it would help to talk to someone who has some experience of this sort of thing.'

And so we did, and as could have been expected, she came that very same day. It was almost four years since we had seen her, yet we had come to know her so well that it did not seem so. Except that she was a little stouter now, there was no change in the calm and kindly, sensitive and sensible person that she was. We told her the whole story—of our search for alternatives, of our fears about Haughton, and about keeping her at home. And as always Miss Fraser listened attentively and heard us out. And then she said very much what Martin had already said, only it gave us both more confidence to hear her say it.

And so Lucy went to Haughton.

Chapter 12

IT WAS VERY hard in the early days after Lucy had gone to Haughton, to face the fact that she had joined that horde of pathetic people. Would she become one of them? It was obvious to anyone that Lucy had not suffered by being away at Beechwood. On the contrary, she had been so extremely well-cared-for in every respect that she may well have benefited; but I could not feel confident that she would receive the same care at Haughton.

We had let her go because under all the circumstances that seemed the right thing. But squaring it with one's conscience was another matter. It was one thing to tell people she was at Beechwood, quite another to let them know she was at Haughton. How could anyone believe we loved her, and yet had allowed her to go there?

I had always felt guilty about sending Lucy away, and was always on the defensive, always feeling I had to give reasons and offer explanations. I was very conscious of the unspoken criticism of society. A mother, society says, who gives up the daily care of her child, is a bad mother; one to be blamed, not pitied. So often when I told people their faces assumed a mask and they turned away. What could I say? I needed a whole hour to explain all the reasons that would justify my action. And most people had no time or desire for that. I got the impression that people condemned us without ever knowing or caring about the circumstances. So much easier to run one's life on a pre-packed set of cliché values, cliché judgements, cliché principles, and cliché emotions. But perhaps it was my uneasy conscience which coloured my reading of their disinterest.

Unable to excuse myself to people, I railed in my notebook again:

My baby is a mongol. No one in this enlightened age will blame me for that; but we have sent her away to an institution, and that no one can condone. It still, apparently, needs to be said, that no mother parts with her baby painlessly; it is a hard thing to do—more especially so in this new modern climate of optimism and hope, when all the social and economic pressures are towards leaving such children with their families. Society abhors the idea of shutting away idiots in dark Victorian institutions, so leave her at home. Everywhere they are opening bright newly-designed Day Training Centres, lavishly equipped, and staffed by crusaders, so leave her at home. Everyone deplores the idea of a mother rejecting her child, of a family rejecting one of its members, so shoulder the burden, don't count the cost, don't think about ten years hence, just leave her at home. But we didn't, and the cross of the knowledge of her environment now is a heavier one than that other, for me. But I was the sister of a handicapped child, and I learned things to which you will not listen.

I had started supply teaching about a year before, and was now to begin a permanent full-time post. I had tried hard to get a job with handicapped children, but there were no special schools in my area, nor any peripatetic work. I was sorry about that. Although I enjoyed teaching normal children, and found it satisfying and stimulating, yet I wanted to be of service to the handicapped. I felt my experience could have been helpful in an area where there was plenty of need for help, but, more than that, being of service to the handicapped generally would have salved my conscience a little about Lucy. Surely I would be more use to the community teaching a classful of handicapped children, than by spending all my life-energy and spirit nursing just one at home?

I threw myself into my job and tried to put Lucy out of my mind. But I had to visit her—how easy it would have been not to. And after all the nightmares I had suffered remembering that array of blank faces, it did not seem anything like so horrifying when I went again.

Lucy was in a small special-care ward for young children, many of whom were bed-ridden. But there was a small play-room for mobile children like Lucy, and I found her playing quite happily in a group. I had come alone so that Martin could stay with Julia, and I took Lucy out in the car. We stopped in the countryside where I had tea from a flask, and Lucy had a tin of sieved fruit which she was accustomed to having at Beechwood. We went for a walk and we played. I watched her critically. Was she well? Was she happy? Was she quite as bright as she always was before? She seemed so, and I was very relieved. I had not realized till then how screwed up with anxiety I had been.

I took her back to the ward, which, though rather bare, yet had a good many toys in the play-room and in the cots, and the nurses seemed young and affable. I left a number of tins of sieved fruit and a bottle of blackcurrant juice, and asked if she could have them, and they said that she could. I looked around for her own dolls but could not see them. However, I told myself, since Lucy does not really know them, it won't matter to her, so long as there are toys to play with. She was not wearing her own clothes either, though she had plenty and that too, I thought, won't matter to her so long as she is adequately clothed.

I kissed her and turned to go, waving goodbye. She smiled up at me and waved too—the last thing she had learned to do at Beechwood.

I went to sister's office and spoke to her. She assured me that Lucy had settled in well and that there were no problems. Lucy, she said, was not quite ready to attend the school yet, nor to be with the older fully mobile children, but she would be going as soon as she was able.

I looked through the window as I left, and saw Lucy quite happily engrossed with a toy, the other children around her, and I came away content.

We fell into a pattern of visiting. Because of the distance we could not see her as frequently as before, but we went about once a month and phoned weekly. Usually I went alone on a Saturday or a Sunday, and Martin stayed with Julia. Julia was at school all the week, and, because of his erratic working hours, Martin was often not there to see her in the evenings, nor for the week-end. His time with her was so limited therefore that we thought it best for him to stay with her on those days when I visited Lucy. I was glad that he did. The return journey and the time spent with Lucy took up most of the day, and I did not want Julia, still so insecure, parked out for so long. This way I could go without being anxious about her.

I cannot remember exactly when it was that we first began to feel concerned about Lucy. I think we really became worried when she came home for Christmas. I had noticed earlier that she was looking thinner and had mentioned it to sister, but she was not concerned about it, saying that Lucy was too plump before. But at home I could see that as well as having lost a little weight, Lucy was less lively than she always had been. Mother said she thought Lucy's behaviour was improving—she was less destructive, less boisterous, more amenable than before. Mother thought she was simply growing up—but I was not so sure.

She did not eat with such gusto as before, and even had to be fed and coaxed again. When we went to the Boxing Day hunt she seemed to feel the cold, and lolled feebly against Martin as he carried her. Her nappies too were a greater problem. She had never had any control at all, but now we had much looser messes, more often. But she played happily enough at home in the warm, and kept us all very busy rushing around after her.

I spoke to sister about it when we took her back. She was sure that there was nothing really wrong, but said she would ask the doctor to examine her on his next round. When I phoned later she said the doctor was quite satisfied with Lucy, and that she was to be moved into a children's cottage, from which she would attend morning school. I was pleased to hear this because I thought that she would enjoy the school.

Anxious about her I began to visit more frequently. She did not, at first, seem unhappy—but she was not the bright person-ality she was. The new 'cottage' seemed much less well-run than the one Lucy had left. There was a great number of children of all ages together in one big room. They seemed lively enough from what one could see of them, but that was very little. Always when one went one was kept well away from the room which served as dining- and play-room. There was a small reception room with a bell, where visitors were expected to wait for their children to be brought to them. Often I was worried by the long wait. Whatever did they have to do to her before they fetched her just that few yards? If one did see another child in the corridor it was likely to be without socks or shoes, or without knickers.

I began to find an occasional bruise or two on her face or her arms, but when I asked how she got them, the staff never knew. Always the nurse on duty had come to the ward only that morning; always the sister was off-duty or somewhere else or otherwise unavailable. The staff seemed to be constantly moving around to the numerous other wards, and no one ever knew anything.

She came home again at Easter, and we were alarmed to discover that she had lost more weight. And now it was obvious that she was less active. She would sit quietly in an armchair and hardly move for a long time and it seemed clear to me that something was wrong. Yet still Mother and neighbours and relatives who saw her insisted that she seemed quite all right. 'She is just growing up,' they said, 'calming down a little. It's a very good thing that she is. She was quite uncontrollable before.' Martin was not so sure—like me, he was uneasy.

When I took her back I intended to see the ward sister, but as usual she was not there. I asked to see the doctor, but that was not possible. I said I would make an appointment to come up to see them both, but it seemed that I could not do that either. I left the ward then and went to the adminstrative block, determined to see someone about it. But there was no one to see, only a few office girls who said that if I wished to see the superintendent I should write for an appointment.

I wrote for an appointment, suggesting a time and date, and since I had no reply to my letter assumed that the time was convenient. But when I arrived I was not expected, and neither the superintendent nor any other doctor had prepared to see me. I was passed along a chain of office girls and helpers of various kinds until I ended up in a sort of over-crowded office with someone who said he was the assistant to the superintendent. Blandly he assured ne that the doctor would see her, that he would ask for a report, that all would be well; but I went away uneasy.

When I visited Lucy a week later I was told that the doctor had seen Lucy, and had prescribed iron tablets because she was anaemic. She had more bruises on her face and her arms and again, no one knew anything about them.

We were deeply worried by this time, about her health, and about the apparent lack of care and concern. We began to fetch her home for an occasional weekend, and to visit her every week. When I visited I drove her out to a quiet part of the estate where I could undress her to check her body for bruises or marks. I began to notice, regularly, that there were little pin-prick bruises at the top of her arms, and assumed that she was having injections, but when I asked the nurses about it they assured me that she was not. On one occasion she had lost a finger-nail, but no one knew how. Though I pursued it I never discovered the cause.

As I left, my eyes flooded with unspilt tears, one of the older women patients who came to the ward to help with the children, ran out after me, and seeing my tears, she put her arms around me unselfconsciously, and comforted me saying, 'Don't you worry about Lucy, I'll look after her. I love Lucy. I'll look after her.'

She was as dishevelled as any, her face lined and wrinkled, her speech thick and slurred and difficult to understand, but her perception and concern for my feelings was touching, and her affection for Lucy was warm and real, and I was humbly grateful to her.

Eventually I saw sister again and tried to impress upon her how concerned I was about Lucy's weight loss, and she promised to keep a special eye on her. When I next visited she came out to see me, smiling serenely, convinced that she had discovered the reason. Lucy, she said, had been sitting at a table with bigger and more assertive children who had been taking her food. Now she had moved Lucy to another table with children who were fed by the helpers, and she was sure all would now be well!

It was a painful time for us all. Working all the week, and making the long drive to Haughton most weekends, or fetching Lucy home, and then always fretting about her between visits, I was becoming very difficult to live with—and saw little of Julia. More and more Martin took over the care of Julia, while I became totally preoccupied with Lucy again. There was no time now in Martin's life for anything other than work and household chores.

Julia began to resist going to school and pleaded to stay away. Wendy had moved away a few months before and Julia had made no other friends. Other girls, she said, called her names and jeered at her in the play-ground. She began to fret about her classwork too, being always confused and worried about what precisely she should be doing. A good deal of her work seemed to involve cutting and sticking and drawing pictures, and since she was not a dexterous child, the effort involved and the messy work she produced, made her miserably conscious of her shortcomings.

Often she challenged us to explain to her why she had to go to school, and when we told her that she had to learn, she would say 'But what is it that I'm learning at school that I couldn't learn from a book at the library?' and it was hard to answer her arguments.

We fetched Lucy home as soon as my school-holidays began. There was no question now that she was ailing. She was becoming more and more apathetic, hardly moving or taking much interest in anything around her.

Again we wrote for an appointment to see the superintendent, and this time followed it up with a phone-call the next day. Although it seemed that it was impossible to see the superintendent, it was possible to see a doctor.

We both went up to see him, and were surprised at the small dingy office, obviously shared by two others. The doctor was a quiet and anxious man who listened seriously to what we had to say. He spent a long time looking at Lucy's papers and thinking about it. Yes, he said, they did have a note about her weight loss; yes, she had been given iron for her anaemia. He was obviously concerned, but at a loss to know what to do about it. He spoke of the difficulties, the great number of real medical problems for such a small team to deal with; the impossibility of getting reliable information from the wards because they had too few nurses, most of them untrained, all over-worked.

He seemed quite overwhelmed by the practical difficulties; but they did he said, have their own hospital block there, and the obvious thing to do would be to take her in for a few days' observation. The only problem was that the hospital was permanently filled with older chronic bed-ridden patients, and it was difficult to find a bed for any other. But he said he would make every effort to do that the very next week.

So we left Lucy at Haughton then while we went for a holiday ourselves. We stayed with Martin's sister in Devon, where Julia had cousins to play with, but for me it was a misery, being separated from Lucy when she obviously needed me.

We went to fetch her home again as soon as we got back, and learned that she had not been in the hospital after all, because there was no vacant bed. The only thing to do, the young nurse on duty told us, was to wait until someone in the hospital died. We noticed, even as we stood there talking to the nurse and holding Lucy, that she appeared to be running a temperature, but the nurse thought that Lucy was hot from sitting in the sun, and praised her for being so 'good'.

Even in the short time that we were away she seemed to me to have deteriorated. It seemed too, as if it was more than just a reluctance to eat. She would take food to her mouth and swallow, but then would cry feebly as if it hurt her. She had lost a little more weight and was almost completely passive, sitting propped in a chair or lying on the sofa for long periods without moving, and crying a little when she was disturbed.

We called our own new doctor up to see her, but he was not convinced that there was anything wrong with her. 'Lots of children,' he said, 'are very thin without being ill, and mongols often do become more passive as they get older.' I told him what an increased problem the nappies were. In fact, nappies would not contain her messes any more, which oozed out everywhere.

She needed several bathes a day. But Dr Miller thought that was only natural, since she was now nearly six. Still it seemed to me that it was very unnatural.

The end of my holidays drew near. I had nursed and fed her for several weeks and she was no better; she was, in fact, rather worse. I had called in my own doctor and he could find nothing wrong with her. What was the next step now?

I could not think what I ought to do, I only knew what I wanted to do: that was to keep her at home and continue to nurse her. I longed to have her with me, to give up my job and just tend her. At least I could keep her warm and comfortable. I yearned for that from the deepest core of my being.

I spoke of it to Martin, but even before I spoke I knew what his response would be. He would appeal to my reason and tell me that Lucy must go back to Haughton, and I must go back to teaching. I sensed, and understood and shared at heart, the fears he had about keeping Lucy at home. We both knew that once we gave up Lucy's place, she was never likely to be offered another, and we saw that as a threat, not only to Lucy, but to the family.

Martin had been shocked when he had come to realize how much Julia had been affected by that first year. He shared my guilt about that, and my fear that all her remaining childhood years were not enough to repair the harm we had done to her then. And Martin feared for me too. The years when Lucy had been at Beechwood had been a time of spiritual and emotional recuperation for us—we had restored our souls again. Now Martin was trying very hard not to let this experience of Lucy at Haughton threaten the family again.

So often he tried to comfort me. 'She may be very passive', he said, 'but just look at her. She is quite happy. She wants nothing. She will never suffer as you and I and Julia have suffered.

'Oh, yes, I know that all your criticisms of Haughton are just. But all these details which worry you, do not affect Lucy greatly, and no good—no long-term good—for her or us, will come from simply bringing her home.'

'Make as much fuss as you like—do what you can to change

things—but you are only in a position to do that while Lucy is there.'

And in my heart I knew he was right. So Lucy went back to Haughton, and I started a new term.

Chapter 13

THE WEEKS THAT followed were strained and tense. I began to find it hard to concentrate on my school work. Previously in my life, teaching had been a very separate compartment. I had been able to tune in and out of school- or family- self, and once tuned into school, or at least, once inside the class-room, all else in my personal life was shut out and I became wholly absorbed.

But this switching became more and more difficult, and often I could not achieve it. My work began to suffer—though at first no one noticed it but me. I was able to draw on past experience, repeat lessons I had planned and thought out long before, respond from habit rather than new appraisal. For some time I could continue on the momentum I had gathered previously.

I began to brood a great deal about Lucy's symptoms. I continued to see her frequently, and as time went by her body resumed the shape it had been in the first year of her life—a vast distended abdomen and thin twig-like limbs. At first I thought it was the receding chest and the diminishing limbs which emphasized the abdomen again, but suddenly it occured to me that that too might be a symptom of whatever was wrong with her.

I went to the library again and looked up the medical books. I came across an illness I had not heard of before—coeliac disease —whose symptoms exactly coincided with Lucy's. It meant that the sufferer was not able to digest gluten, an ingredient of wheat, and consequently of anything containing wheat-flour, and if it was not removed from the diet would have a poisoning effect.

Could it really be this? Or something like it? Had I found a clue?

I made another appointment to see the doctor, but when I

arrived it was a different doctor. He too, seemed worried and tired. He had a slight speech impediment and a limp, and, like the other, he went slowly and carefully through Lucy's file.

I told him how much more pronounced now were all the symptoms I had noticed earlier, and he agreed that it was so. He said that Lucy had been taken out of school now, and left in bed on the ward in the mornings, since she seemed too weak to cope with a whole day up. He, too, spoke of the difficulties of making a diagnosis.

Hesitantly, tentatively, mildly,—knowing on what unstable ground a lay-person stood, who suggested a diagnosis to a doctor—I asked, could it possibly be coeliac disease? He seemed a little suprised at my question, but said yes, they had considered the possibility themselves, and had tried to test for it, but had some difficulty. It was, he said, necessary to collect all the stools for twenty-four hours, but conditions on the wards were such that they could not be sure that they were given all, nor even that all they were given were in fact hers. I was shocked, but equally it was obvious that he himself was deeply troubled by the situation.

My pity then went out to him, and to the others like him there who were working against such odds. What chance did they have? How soul-destroying for them to be in such a situation. No wonder they were short of doctors! What reward was there for them here?

But he was going on. He would, he said, try to get her put on to a diet which excluded or at least reduced the amount of bread and biscuits, though, he said, it was very difficult to keep one child on a diet in these circumstances.

I felt humbled by his concern, and by his desire to go on under the appalling circumstances of his work. He must, I thought, be truly dedicated.

But I was concerned for Lucy. 'If conditions here,' I said, 'are such that you cannot adequately treat Lucy, is it possible that she could be transferred to an ordinary hospital?' 'That would be best for her,' he agreed, 'but we cannot do that. You see, technically we are a hospital ourselves, so we cannot transfer our patients; and if we started sending all our medical problems to the local hospitals, we should very soon swamp them.' I went back out to the car and wept then, and I wept while I was driving most of the sixty miles home.

It was becoming quite impossible to carry on with my job. The mornings I coped with, but as soon as we stopped for the lunchtime break, I broke down and sobbed on my desk in the privacy of my class-room. Lunchtimes were always the hardest to endure, especially if I got into the car to do some shopping. Once behind the driving wheel I was seized by the urge to drive out of the town and on to Haughton to collect Lucy and go away with her. Just she and I away—to retreat from family and school and the problems of my present life. But where? And how could I possibly leave Martin and Julia? It was a foolish game my mind was playing—toying with the idea of leaving Martin and Julia for Lucy.

All the painful months and years since Lucy's birth Martin and I had clung to each other. All the most hopeless moments we had shared together: we had comforted and supported each other, alone against an alien world. Hurt as each of us was, we had both been deeply concerned for each other, and for Julia and Lucy. Now I felt that the years had worn us down, and were turning us in different ways. We could sustain each other no longer.

Julia was increasingly unhappy at school. She worried excessively because she could not thread her needle, or jump off the apparatus, or had no partner for dancing. She was too afraid to go to the cloakroom alone, too timid to ask anyone to go with her. When I fetched her from school she was solemn and silent, standing apart from the others, much as our traumatized hen had done.

It was obvious that I could not carry on teaching in my emotional state. But Martin was anxious that I should not blot my teaching career by collapsing in mid-term, so he persuaded me to see my headmaster and give notice to leave at Christmas. The proper date for notice had gone by, but my headmaster was sympathetic about the situation and agreed that I should go. Poor man, he was probably quite relieved to be rid of me.

I went to see my own doctor, seeking further advice about Lucy—but he only gave me tranquillizers, and insisted on making an appointment for me to see a psychiatrist. He could make no suggestion as to what I could do about Lucy.

When next I visited Lucy I was appalled to see her new bruises. She had a large regular bruise between her eyes, and the eyes were bloodshot; two equally regular bruises were on either side of her face, just below the temples, and she had another just below her chin. It was a horrifying sight—and seemed to suggest that she had been encased in some sinister medieval torture instrument.

Everyone on the ward gave me a different explanation, and each one a more transparent fabrication than the last. They looked at each other shiftily when I insisted on seeing the doctor.

'Yes,' he said, regretfully when I asked, Lucy had been attacked by another patient. Unhappily he had now had to put the patient under heavy sedation in the hospital block. He was obviously deeply disturbed about the incident. 'Occasionally,' he said, 'a patient will become violent. What is one to do? It is quite impossible to keep them isolated or under heavy sedation all the time.'

I left then, and from a public phone-box called the office of the county medical officer, and asked for an appointment to see him, or his deputy in charge of services for the handicapped. 'Oh, that will be Miss Mason you want to see,' she said, and I recognized the name of the young psychologist who had first seen Lucy five years ago. 'When would you like to come?' I said it was rather urgent and if it were at all possible I should like to come that day. It was possible and I drove straight there.

I told her all about it; about Lucy ailing, and growing too weak to be up all day; about the appalling conditions at Haughton and the impossibility of her getting adequate treatment; about this last attack and how many times before I had suspected something like this.

She listened, but she was not shocked as anyone should have been. Like my own doctor, she seemed to think it was just a matter of my pining for Lucy, and did not seem to give much credence to my report of conditions there. I tried to point out that I had been perfectly happy separated from Lucy when she was well-cared-for at Beechwood, but Miss Mason was not impressed. 'Have you been to see the superintendent about all this?' she asked. 'Have you', I parried, 'had an audience with the queen? It would be easier to arrange than an audience with the superintendent of Haughton.' 'Have you seen your own doctor?' she said. 'He would be able to give you some tranquillizers.' 'What I need', I screamed at her, 'is proper provision for my daughter. Not drugs to make me accept conditions that should never be accepted.'

That same medical service which had been so concerned for Lucy's survival when she was a baby, cared little about her now. Suffering, it seems, is relatively unimportant. The quality of life counts for nothing—only death, or the threat of it, makes an impact.

Martin was aghast when I told him about the attack on Lucy, and appalled at hearing of the indifference of the county medical staff. And he too, became, like me, more concerned for Lucy's immediate comfort than for long-term considerations for the family, and he agreed that, if we were not able to get Lucy transferred to a more satisfactory hospital or home by the time I finished teaching at Christmas, then we should keep her at home. It was a decision we both recognized as a defeat.

I kept the appointment with the psychiatrist and answered his questions honestly, and told him about Lucy. 'Well,' he said after about an hour and a half, 'I can't think why they sent you to me. It seems to me that your unstable emotional state is a very reasonable response to a stressful situation. The cure for that is to remove the stress by getting something done about your daughter. I shall send your doctor a report to that effect.'

As I was leaving and thanking him, he came and whispered confidentially, 'By the way, next time you have your daughter home for a few days, call your own doctor up to see her again. If he thought she was ill, he might be able to get her into an ordinary hospital—if he was prepared to stick his neck out a bit.'

We fetched Lucy home the next weekend, and I asked for a

few days off school to lengthen her stay. She was already running a temperature when we fetched her, so we called Dr Miller up that evening. He called the next day, and the next, and on the third visit he said, 'Well, it does seem that there is something very wrong with her—I'll see if I can get her seen by a specialist at the Great Ormond Street Hospital for Sick Children.'

Dutifully we took her back to Haughton. She cried feebly when we arrived. Was she crying with the pain in her tummy, or did she recognize her surroundings and fear to go in? Never before had she given any positive sign of recognizing a place, or shown any reluctance to go anywhere. But I knew that it would only be for a few weeks longer, so I steeled myself and we took her in.

We had a letter within a few days giving us an appointment for Lucy to be seen at the out-patients' department of the Great Ormond Street Hospital.

We all went up to London together and Martin took Julia off to the Natural History Museum to pay homage to the Blue Whale, as on our rare visits to London he always did. Martin was trying very hard to keep up normal family activities with Julia, and to shield her from the anxieties we felt.

At the hospital I took Lucy first to be weighed and measured. The nurse put her on the scales, but she swayed and tottered so much that they had to put her in the chair-scales. They stood her up against the measuring rod, but her knees buckled and her head lolled. I had to hold her knees straight, and a nurse her head, so that they could gauge her height.

She was seen by an elderly, kind, and gentle specialist who agreed that she should go in as soon as they had a vacant bed.

We had a letter shortly afterwards to say that she could go a few days after Christmas.

I wrote to Haughton to tell them that Lucy was going into the Great Ormond Street Hospital and in some trepidation awaited their response. After all, I was really, I supposed, going behind their backs, and wasn't quite sure of the ethics of it. But I need not have worried. Their response was exactly the same as always—that is, there was no response at all.

I never did see the superintendent.

Chapter 14

WE FETCHED LUCY home a few days before Christmas and her sixth birthday. I was light-headed with relief, with the positive joy of feeling that something was to be done at last.

It was a subdued Christmas. We went through the usual family rituals, but Lucy needed nursing and after the past months of anxiety it was a luxury to be able to indulge my instinct to tend her.

She spent most of the holiday lying propped on the settee. Her round eyes followed Julia whenever she came into range, but she seemed too weak and listless to turn her head. Frequently she fell asleep, and waking again would still lie passively against the cushions, rarely finding sufficient energy to get up and play with Julia. When Christmas was over I was glad to be able to drop the pretence of feeling festive.

We braced ourselves for the next ordeal—taking Lucy to Great Ormond Street. She, listless, hardly noticed the journey, and seemed quite unmoved by her new surroundings when she arrived. Sister and a young nurse came over to help Lucy settle in bed. We discussed whether she would be better in a cot or a bed, and decided on a cot. I attached her cradle-play and her soft toys to the bars—all new because the old ones had not been returned from Haughton—and after the form filling, and an interview with the young houseman, I was invited to bath and feed Lucy myself before leaving her.

The ward was broken up into small bays and cubicles, and Lucy was in a room for four. It seemed light and bright, with lots of bustle—children careering down the passages on tricycles, nurses with noisy trays of jostling bottles, teachers and therapists and mums by bedsides, and a diversity of cheerful white-coated medical staff and students, which made the ward about as busy as Piccadilly Circus. Lots to interest, to stimulate, to reassure a frightened child—a great contrast to the stagnant atmosphere at Haughton. Certainly, it reassured me. So many nurses. And all so young and alert, and all so ready to smile and pat and chat to the children as they passed.

A number of older children came over to greet Lucy, and a number of mums and nurses and voluntary workers chatted to me. Whatever was wrong with Lucy, I had every confidence that here it would be diagnosed and treated.

It was with relief that I wept on this drive home. Martin was silent, intent on negotiating the traffic, but I could feel his mood in tune with my own—the enormous sense of release from the months of emotional turmoil. We held hands whenever we paused for traffic, and comfort flowed between us.

Julia had spent the day alone with Mother, and she was quiet when we arrived home. She stared hard at my red bulging eyes, but already was restrained enough not to comment—or perhaps, after the number of times she had seen me like that in the last few months, it was no longer a subject for comment or question. I hugged her to me, guilty and regretful at what my own perpetual misery must be doing to her.

I went up to see Lucy a week later. She seemed placid and happy and was even sitting up in her cot, watching the comings and goings, and listening to the music. Sister and nurses all made much of her, and everyone seemed especially fond of her. When I spoke to the doctor he was reluctant to say much, preferring to wait for the results of tests they had made.

I went down, at his suggestion, to see one of the hospital's own social workers, and told her about Lucy's previous unhappy situation. Immediately she said she would make enquiries about finding an alternative place for Lucy when she was discharged. She pointed out that the average length of stay in Great Ormond Street was ten days, though she thought that it might be a bit longer than this in Lucy's case. She seemed hopeful that she might find a better long-term place for Lucy, and the joy of hope sang in my head again. Perhaps, after all, a place might be found for Lucy where she could be as happy and as well cared for as

age-range from five to seventeen, an
have had in a permanent post. As I
yself called upon more and more, until
eral places at once.

ster I had a visit from the county edu-
ith handicapped children. He had come
ffices especially to see me 'unofficially'.
a vacant post in my area for a peripa-
Had I seen the advertisement? Would
for it? He went on to say that the post
would be an extra salary allowance for
ldren, another because it was a post of
ar and mileage allowance. It would be
should be visiting the few deaf children,
ide rural area, who were too young yet
o for various other reasons, sometimes
t in a special school or unit.

post I had always dreamed of. I should
have been able to accept it—but how
hen we had found no place for Lucy? I
d he saw how regretful I was to have to
t the post had been advertised several
ad had not a single suitably qualified
he shortage of teachers for the deaf.
it, and he said that for the sake of those
eady been without a teacher for so long
rmanent teacher, but should he be un
me to me again, and he hoped that
et Lucy a place which would leave
'Surely,' he said incredulously, 'sure
oyed teaching these deaf children, th
nd your one little mongol.' Even
with work for the handicapped, c
situation regarding provision for
as in such a critical state.
about it he was surprised and pl
wanted very much to be able to ta

she had been at Beechwood. The world looked bright and full of colour again. It had been a dim grey for so long.

When I went the next week the doctor gave me his diagnosis. Lucy, on admission, had been suffering from a collapsed left lung, a rare intestinal infection called giardia, and coeliac disease, which, having been untreated for so long, had caused a considerable amount of damage to the gut.

The collapsed lung was apparently already responding to treatment, and the giardia taken care of by antibiotics. But the coeliac and the gut damage would require longer treatment. She had been put on a diet which excluded anything containing gluten or sugars of any kind, including lactose and fructose. This meant excluding everything containing flour, sugar, milk, butter, most fruit and certain vegetables. It would have been a very limited diet indeed but for their special facilities for dealing with it. The doctor was hopeful that Lucy would, in time, respond to diet, though they might have to experiment a bit with various foods; and the gut should heal when it was no longer being irritated.

He assured me that Lucy would recover, and begin to make progress again when she was established on a diet that she could tolerate, but he warned that her stay there might have to be measured in months rather than weeks. He urged me to see his social worker again to check on progress about finding Lucy an alternative long-stay place when they had to discharge her.

Lucy did slowly make progress. Each time I saw her she seemed a little more alert and active. There came an occasion only a few weeks later when I was distressed to see her standing up in her cot in a restraining harness. Apparently she had become so much more lively that, not only did she stand in her cot but was constantly trying to climb out, and on one accasion succeeded. She was now, sister assured me, taken out of her cot for a period every morning and afternoon, but while she was in it, it was not safe to leave her without a harness.

She cried when I left. I think it was the first time that she had ever done that. My heart was heavy at seeing her distress, and I wondered what it indicated for the future.

She cried when we left at the next visit too, when Martin and Julia were with me, and Julia was very upset at seeing her cry. She was puzzled too at seeing Martin and I walk firmly away. Outside the door she urged us to go back. 'Mummy, Daddy, why don't you go back and stop Lucy crying? Why is she crying Mummy? Does she want to come home?' Lucy cried so rarely, but when she did it was the most heart-rending sight and sound in the world. How could we turn our backs and walk away? We loitered outside the ward and tried to see her through the windows to reassure ourselves.

At the next visit we found her happily brushing the rug-wool hair of the floppy rag-doll that Julia had made for her, and she did not cry again.

My visits to Great Ormond Street were very different from my visits to Haughton. Here I was quite free to bath and feed Lucy, to play with her on the floor, to walk her along to the playroom. At Haughton one was simply expected to remove the child from the ward regardless of the weather, and was not free to share any of the child's usual activities.

Here I spoke freely to the many nurses and other staff around —indeed if I did not they quickly approached me with some anecdote of Lucy's latest mischief. At Haughton the staff seemed to avoid visiting parents, and if approached, rarely had any personal knowledge of one's own child.

It was a very different child I visited after a month or so. She was up for longer periods and was walking along to the day-room for her meals where she sat at a table with other children and fed herself, wielding her spoon and fork deftly and cleanly. And soon she would come running along the corridor to meet me when I arrived, and would see me off at the door trundling a wooden horse, and would leave me happily to trundle it back again when I left. Her progress medically may not have been especially impressive, but the progress she made personality-wise was truly amazing. The combination of improving health and vitality, and a friendly encouraging environment, made her blossom again like the blackthorn after the winter.

I continued to see the social worker at intervals, and she wa

post, both for the work itself, which I knew I could do, and because the feeling that I was of some value to the community
would help to assuage those feelings of guilt I always had about
Lucy being away. It would, as it were, cancel my debt to society.

But in the meantime Lucy was still at Great Ormond Street.
She was making good progress, and we waited, expecting each
week to hear that she would soon be discharged.

And then in May the doctor said that they thought it a good
idea to send Lucy across to the psychiatric hospital across the
road to have her intelligence and her future potential assessed.
Of course we agreed. She had made great progress in recent
months, both socially and physically, and we hoped the prog-
nosis might be a little better, And yet, in conflict again, I felt
too that Lucy was happy now, as she was, and with future care
and a sympathetic environment would always be. To be a few
points further up the IQ scale, to be able to be trained to do this
or that would not necessarily make her happier or more satisfied
with herself, would it? I waited uneasily, not sure what I hoped
the result would be.

Lucy was assessed as profoundly subnormal. She was not
expected to develop a great deal more than she had already.
She was unlikely to acquire speech, at least not more than a few
words at most; she might develop some bowel or bladder control later on, but might not; she should learn to dress herself
with help but would never learn the fears and inhibitions and
restraints of a normal child, and would need constant supervision
always. She would always be happy providing that she was well
cared for.

It came as a relief not to have to hope, to imagine, to antici-
pate, what Lucy would be like in later years. She would be much
as she was now—happy, mischievous, and affectionate—who
could worry about that? How much more worrying to be the
parent of a border-line child, one who might just cope, or might
not; one for whom the future was doubtful, whose place in
society was precarious. And how much more painful for the child
himself, who might discern his own limitations? Lucy never
would.

Julia too had her intelligence assessed when we took her back to the Child Guidance Clinic because of her difficulties at school. She broke their highest norm, and her IQ was stated as 170 plus.

What a strange irony of fate! Lucy's IQ was about 30, so if you could have mixed the two children together and rolled them out again like gingerbread-men, we would have had two average children—as indeed statistically we had. No wonder she was finding it difficult to fit in—she was as far removed from most of her age-peers as Lucy was.

It did in some measure explain the difficulties she experienced at school. Insecure and highly suggestible as she was, she had become confused and more unsure of herself when she saw her class-mates struggle with things which had been apparently clear to her for years. Her natural shyness and timidity made her reluctant to be distinguished from the group in any way—she was as fearful of praise as of blame, as reluctant to be 'top' as 'bottom'—and strove always to conform to the common pattern of behaviour and performance, which was as unnatural to her as to Lucy.

Her own image of herself deteriorated as she became aware that she did not match up to the ideals of the group, did not share their attitudes to people, to learning, to life. She was always different because she was always at a different stage of development, and in any group of children—almost any society—the greatest crime is to be different. In this she shared the affliction of her sister; both deviated from the usual norm of intelligence—but Julia must live in society, Lucy never would.

At school she was moved to a class of children a year older, and she did have much more in common with them in interest and outlook. The work she took easily in her stride except for things like needlework and ball games.

In her new class Julia did slowly gain enough confidence to enable her to cope with school, and she did find another friend—an intelligent, introverted and sensitive girl who is her friend still.

Julia had some early success as a writer. She wrote a piece which was entered for a literary competition—and won. Subsequently it was published and broadcast several times in this and other countries. Any child might have been pleased, but Julia was only embarrassed. By the time it appeared in print her ideas had already moved on, and she regarded it as 'babyish'.

In June a young American houseman on an exchange at the hospital for a short time disturbed me very much. He had wanted he said, to give Lucy a chromosome count. This, he explained, would establish beyond doubt whether in fact she was a mongol or not. 'A little trisome,' he called her. Apparently she should have one extra chromosome, and until this were ascertained in a laboratory test one could not be absolutely certain of her condition. He explained that in his hospital in the US every suspected case had this test as a matter of course, to rule out the possibility of any other condition, which might give rise to similar symptoms, but which was remediable.

Lucy had never been tested, and the consultant here, he explained, thought there was little point in having an expensive test which could only confirm the obvious. The young American asked what I felt about it, but I could not give him a coherent answer—I was so agitated by the merest suggestion that there could be any doubt.

My God, was it possible? Was there even a one-in-a-million chance that after all she was not a mongol? That she was instead suffering some condition that could have been treated in babyhood? The very mention of the possibility threw me into a turmoil. If it were proved now to have been a mistaken diagnosis how could I bear it?

I was in a panic. 'No, no,' I shouted at him, 'I don't want her tested now. It's six years too late.' And so, to my knowledge, she never was.

It was about this time that Lucy was 'borrowed' by the medical school near-by to be used as a model for the medical-students' examinations. For this she was paid the usual fee of ten shillings. Sister handed it to me sealed in an envelope with Lucy's name on it. Embarrassed, I handed it back to her suggesting that she got some flowers for the ward, but briskly she refused to take it, saying that it was Lucy's money—she had earned it. I was deeply touched and impressed. To think that such a helpless dependent little scrap could actually 'earn' money. We bought her a Premium Bond with a chance that it might one day bring her much more.

The hospital social worker had first offered hopefully to find Lucy an alternative long-stay home in the first week of January, and she still had had no success. She herself had been astonished to find the situation quite so bad as it was. There were just no vacant places anywhere, and everywhere had long waiting lists.

As a very last resort she had, without our knowledge, approached Haughton to inform them that Lucy would soon be discharged, but they too refused her—during her absence her place had been taken by another. That particular piece of news did not bother Martin or me because we had agreed that she should not return there, but the staff at Great Ormond Street were highly indignant about it.

It looked as if Lucy would be coming home to live after all, and we resigned ourselves to it.

Lucy was by now up most of the day and was getting daily more energetic and boisterous. It was getting more difficult to cope with her on the ward, to control and restrain her. Lucy would, sister told me, benefit from nursery activities, but she did not fit into their nursery groups. Because she was rather rough they had to keep her with the older children.

The doctor, when I spoke to him, agreed that Lucy would soon be ready to leave. They had not, he said, been able to correct the loose and uncontrolled bowel movements that were the most unpleasant aspect of her condition, but they hoped that her motions would become more normal over the next year or so. Her diet had been modified over the past months, but she was still on a diet which excluded all flour, milk, and dairy produce.

She must, he said, remain on this for several years, possibly for life.

One sunny Saturday afternoon in July shortly before she was to be discharged, I took her out. Sister had packed her in paddi-pads and two pairs of pants, and we went by taxi to St James's Park.

Lucy ran and jumped on the grass happy to be out, and

scattered the pigeons and chased the ducks and ran up, like a friendly puppy, to anyone who came by, holding up her arms to be picked up.

I did not restrain her when she ran up to a couple of young students lying sprawled on the grass, and they responded in a friendly way to her approaches. They were openly curious and wanted to know all about her. Lucy laughed infectiously at a peep-bo game the girl played with her, and I gave my attention to the young man and answered his questions.

He asked me how I had come to know of her condition, and I told him that I must forever be grateful to my doctor for telling me early. It did not seem to be the usual case. Of the mothers of mongols I had met at the Mencaps, almost all had waited many months before being told—in one case a year, in another eighteen months. What cruelty that seemed to me. Those mothers must have suffered a great deal of distress at watching the poor progress of a supposedly normal baby. Usually it was the curious stares of suspicious neighbours which made the anxious mother reject the false assurances of her doctor and finally wrest the true facts from him.

The young man was so interested, and the girl so skilful at keeping Lucy amused, that it was some time before I turned my eyes to her. She was sitting on the young man's white riding mac in a puddle of yellow porridge which oozed from the side of her pants. I whisked her up in my arms, oblivious of the mess I was making of my own clothes, and with burning cheeks mumbled a confused apology and ran off with her.

I had to carry her a long way to the public toilets and we were both well plastered when we arrived. I cleaned us both up as best I could, Lucy chuckling and playing unconcernedly all the while, then with my own clothes quite wet and with Lucy well padded out with most of a toilet roll and held securely in my arms, I made for the nearest road to get a taxi back.

The immediate embarrassment subsided when we both looked clean again and were in the taxi making our getaway—though we still smelled a bit. I wondered how the young couple were coping with their share of it, and how they had reacted to it.

When I had time to consider the significance of it I was very disturbed. This sort of thing had happened often enough in the past—though not usually so publicly—but even though they had warned me, I had not expected it to be quite so bad still. It was going to create quite a few problems in the future.

Chapter 15

Lucy came home early in July, with four foolscap pages of diet instructions and an impressive array of vitamin supplements.

She shouted with joy as we took her in, and stamped across the floor and bounded into a springy armchair to bounce herself up and down—crowing loudly all the time.

Amused at her antics, and pleased to see her so happy, Julia tried to take her hand to lead her round the house. She was eager to show Lucy the bedroom that had been newly prepared for her, the dolls and toys that she herself was passing on to her. But Lucy was happy in her bouncy chair and pushed Julia firmly aside.

I made some tea, confident that Martin would keep an eye fixed on Lucy, and brought it in with the sponge-cake that Julia had made from a packet mix, and with the oat-flapjacks that Julia and Martin together had made up from one of Lucy's special diet recipes.

I put the laden tray down on to the table and suddenly, quick as a flash, Lucy dashed over and with one swift movement, dashed the cups to the floor, and laughed delightedly at the noise of the smashing.

We were all taken aback, and stared for some seconds uncomprehending. Martin recovered first—he was just in time to save the milk and the sugar as Lucy's arm shot out a second time. He picked her up and sat her firmly back in her chair scolding and tapping the back of her hand, but she only laughed and struggled from his grasp and stamped about in the broken china.

It was only with the greatest difficulty that we could restrain her. Small as she was she seemed unusually strong, and was determined to do her own thing. Attempts to restrain her she interpreted as a challenge, a game, and she laughed and

5*

struggled and kicked until she was free. At last I gave in and left the tea-things safely in the kitchen, bringing only my own cup in, while Martin held Lucy on his knee and distracted her attention by play. And then I played with her while Martin retired to the kitchen for his.

This pattern of behaviour persisted. Lucy was so boisterous, so mischievous and uncontrolled, her behaviour so uninhibited, that we could only cope by taking it in turn to amuse and distract her. While I was cooking or washing, Martin had to be every moment with Lucy, and if Martin were in the garden, or taking Julia to the library, I had to have Lucy with me.

She had abounding energy and was hyper-active. Her favourite activity was throwing things, and she would throw anything that was available—shoes, dolls, books, saucepans, fruit, the cat, the mantel-clock or Julia's flower-pots. In the first few days home we had so many things broken that we had to go round the house removing all the ornaments, lamps, flower-vases, and anything movable that was within her reach. We dared not leave a cup or plate about, we had either to hold on to it, or put it right away.

Soon she discovered the sheer delight of bursting a bag of sugar and stamping around in it, and when bags were put out of her reach she would make a lightning grab for the bowl put out on the tea-tray. I learnt to put the shopping away promptly, and Martin put bolts on the kitchen cupboards; but if anything was left unguarded for a moment—sugar, jam, flour, pickles—Lucy would find it, and inevitably would throw, break, and make a lovely mess with it.

We tried securing her in the little chair she had had when she was younger, with a tray that fixed in front to hold her captive, but she soon learned to climb out of it.

And we soon found that it was not wise to leave her in ordinary hard shoes. She kicked about so freely that in self-defence we had to put her in soft slippers.

In the garden she delighted in using her feet to stamp all the plants down. Attracted by Julia working in her own patch of garden one day, she ran over to her and stamped down everything

there. Julia cried about that; she had tried so hard not to cry
when Lucy kicked her, pulled her hair, broke her toys, and tore
her books. 'She doesn't really mean it, Mummy' she would say
to me so often.

Lucy did all this in a spirit of mischief, and simply because she
enjoyed it. She laughed hilariously as she did it, and our frantic
attempts to prevent her, or to clear up the mess in her wake,
only amused her more—it was all one lovely game to Lucy.

That she did enjoy it was glaringly apparent, and indeed,
stamping things down and smashing things is a satisfying
experience—and there was little else that Lucy could do.

We did try smacking her, but with no beneficial effect to any
of us. Both Martin and I were very reluctant—we had to screw
ourselves up to a great pitch to do it—and then Lucy only
laughed at our first attempts. We had to smack her really hard
to make any impression, and then she cried her pathetic cry that
made us all feel so miserable and mean, and as soon as she was
comforted she would get up and repeat her misdoings.

We had been told that she had a mental age of one-and-half to
two years, but that we found to be very misleading. Even though
a normal tot of two years is too young to be reasoned with, yet
already it has developed a great deal of social co-operation and
conformity—just how much is difficult to appreciate until you
have met someone like Lucy, who has not. The two-year-old is
eager to please and quick to learn what forms of behaviour are
disapproved of—Lucy was not.

There was one situation in which Lucy was good—very good.
She loved riding in the car. She would sit and croon to herself
gazing out of the window at the passing scenery and never
seemed to tire of it—going for car rides seemed the only way to
pacify her. And even when we were not going anywhere she was
often so eager to go in the car, that she would sit herself on her
own seat at the back, insist that we do up her harness, and then
sit there rocking backwards and forwards as if pretending she
were on the move. Crooning happily, she would remain there
parked in the courtyard watching the traffic pass on the road. It
was the only time that we had any peace.

The situation was difficult enough when Martin was on his summer leave, but when he returned to work it became heartbreaking. It was quite impossible to supervise and amuse Lucy every moment of the day, and in the few moments of lapsed attention she created chaos.

She scrambled upstairs by herself and stuffed the toilet-roll in the pan, scattered talcum-powder all over the carpet, smeared wet soap on the mirrors, tipped bath-oil on the beds, and turned all the taps on and caused a flood. It was havoc when she got into Julia's room—she upset her models, tore her school-books, and scattered all her treasures.

Sometimes Julia would offer to look after Lucy, but this was of very doubtful value. A thoughtful and gentle nine-year-old was no match for Lucy. Julia loved Lucy and took her own rôle very seriously. Still she wanted Lucy to share her activities, and she would encourage Lucy to do things with her. She did have a degree of success, sometimes keeping Lucy amused for a quarter of an hour or so, but usually it ended in disaster, when Lucy deliberately smashed something or spilt something or struck Julia with something heavy.

When I had to go shopping I tried to take Lucy with me in a harness and reins, since she was getting too big for the pushchair, but she would not walk quietly along the pavement, she tried to make dashes into the road, and when prevented by her reins would simply sit down. Quite often she did this in the middle of a busy road, and when I tried to remedy the situation by pulling her to her feet, she simply lifted her feet off the ground, and tugged and struggled so that it was difficult to control her.

The situation was becoming impossible. We asked Mother to stay, tentatively, apologetically, wondering quite how Mother would endure Lucy's newfound boisterousness—but just having another person around to monitor Lucy's activities would be a help.

Surprisingly Mother coped very well with Lucy. She was getting old and slow herself, and would sit for long periods playing a simple repetitive game like putting marbles back in a box as Lucy took them out. Mother and Lucy would go on and on repeating this sort of action for so long that it would have driven a more alert personality to distraction, but Mother was able to tune in to Lucy's wave-length. Mother did, of course, get tired, and she was quite unable to cope with Lucy in a boisterous mood.

It made a great deal of difference to our lives having Mother there. It left me free for short periods to get on with the endless washing and Lucy's special cooking, and it enabled us to go out sometimes without Lucy—to shop, to take Julia out, or to be alone together ourselves for a few brief precious moments.

Quite often when we returned we found that Lucy had been placated in a bizarre way. Once we founding her finishing off a jar of jam the entire pound of which she had eaten with her fingers. She had jam in her hair, in the folds of her neck, all over her clothes and the table, but it had kept her sitting still and quiet for almost an hour, which was a remarkable feat for Lucy. The ten minutes it took to clean up, and the pound of jam, was a fair exchange for an hour of peace.

Jam was a favourite food of Lucy's especially if it were red. It helped to make palatable much of the hard dry rusk she had. She was allowed few sweets, since they mostly contained either flour or milk-powder.

We worked hard to keep strictly to her diet and maintained a constant vigil to prevent her from eating the many foods she was not allowed, but we were not able, during her numerous escapades, to prevent her from tasting an illicit mouthful of cat-food, detergent powder, bath-oil, and tea-leaves, and she showed a surprising capacity to digest such things without ill-effect. She took her vitamin pills and potions as she did everything else that was edible—enthusiastically. Eating was her greatest pleasure in life.

The 'accident' we had had in St James's Park was repeated frequently around the house, and the bathing and washing and changing this necessitated took up a large part of my time.

Lucy loved her baths—which was fortunate when she needed three or four a day. She would shout and splash and hold on to the handles to swing herself up and down sending gallons of water over the side, but again, the mopping-up was a fair exchange for her few minutes of occupation. Often I would take advantage of her absorption to escape to make the beds or to clean the loo. I knew that while I could hear her shouting and splashing all was well—I need only rush back to check her safety if she became silent.

I continued the attempts I had started on much earlier visits home to teach her to understand a few words. At a certain point in her bath I would need her to stand up so that I could wash her bottom, and I made a point of saying 'Stand up' clearly as I raised her to her feet. After a very long time she came to recognize the spoken word, and to respond by standing up herself, without any help from me. Yet still the response was reserved for that particular situation. If I said 'Stand up' while she was downstairs sitting on the carpet, or in the garden, nothing happened. She would have to be taught to respond to the command in many different situations before she could apply it generally.

I had tried too, over several years, to teach her to say 'more' at meal-times when she wanted a second helping, as she invariably did. One had to be alert to get her attention at just the right moment, between the last spoonful and the dive to some-one else's plate, and then I would point into her bowl and say carefully, 'More,' before giving her another helping. Eventually she did begin to copy me. She would point carefully into her bowl, take a deep breath and make a single-syllable sound—which slowly, over a long period, became an 'm'. As she mouthed her sound, she would give a slow forward nod of her head. Martin and Julia laughed at her imitation of me, obviously I had been giving her another involuntary signal—the nod—which to Lucy was as important a part of the ritual as the sound you had to make.

She learned everything so slowly and laboriously, the stages of learning were so slowed up in her, that it seemed to me that she and others like her would be good subjects for studying the processes of learning, about which we still know so little.

We tried to get Lucy out as much as possible—her love of car-rides, and Martin and Julia's love of the woods tied in very nicely and gave us an opportunity to go out together.

I remember one occasion when we went blackberrying. Martin and Julia went ahead to pick and I stayed with Lucy. She found an interesting pile of fine dust in a tractor rut, and sat down to play in it. I tried to distract her but soon gave up. Tired of spending most of my days restraining her, it seemed easier and wiser to let her play, and rest in the bracken myself.

After some time Martin and Julia were back, and the evening already drawing in, we packed our belongings and set off for the car which was some way away out of sight. Lucy, however, refused to come and went back to her tractor rut again. Being laden with blackberries and picnic things, Martin did not pick her up but went on ahead with Julia. I took Lucy firmly by the arm and attempted to pull her up, but she resisted me with all her strength. I tried persuasion then, calling to her and going on ahead expecting her to follow, but she paid no attention and appeared quite unconcerned. Martin and Julia were already out of sight and I went on a long way and stopped calling, but still she did not come. I hid behind a bush where she could not see me, but she just stayed there all alone in the bracken, unable to see another person or a building, but she was quite happy. If I had left her there I do not think she would have cried until it was from cold or hunger.

As time went by Lucy became more rowdy and I began to wilt under the strain of coping with her. Mother remarked cryptically that really I should stop giving all those vitamins to Lucy and take them myself. But soon Mother herself began to feel the strain and we had to take her back to her own home to rest.

Once again we found ourselves in an intolerable situation. Something just had to be done.

We wrote to the county authority again to ask if, since Lucy had been refused a residential place, she could attend the new day training centre in the next town. We explained the difficulties of tending her at home and her apparent need for training, and we felt hopeful that she would be given a place, travelling daily in the special bus which took other mentally-handicapped from our area.

Our request was promptly refused on three counts. (1) being profoundly subnormal Lucy was not eligible—they had a long waiting-list of 'higher-grade' candidates; (2) they could not take incontinent children; (3) they could not serve special diets at lunchtimes. Lucy was, the letter went on to say, in their opinion the responsibility of the hospital board. We already had a letter from the hospital board saying that she was now the responsibility of the local authority.

It was a severe blow. What were we to do? Could we face years, a life-time of this fevered life—exerting ourselves to the limits simply to constrain Lucy? And what would Lucy be like as she grew bigger and stronger, unless she received some training to conform?

I was indignant at the authorities' refusal to provide for her—as I had been indignant so many times in the past—but now I felt defeated, or at least too despondent to face the long struggle which I knew from experience would lay ahead if we were to persuade the authorities to do something about her. And in the meantime every day was becoming harder than the last. We had to find some remedy ourselves.

The sisters of the local convent ran a small private nursery—all that was left of the school which Julia had attended which had had to close down through lack of funds. I approached the mother superior to ask if Lucy could attend.

Mother Anne was most sympathetic and wanted to help. She was, she said, especially interested in mentally-handicapped children, and being aware of the acute shortage of places for them, had approached the local authority to ask if her school with all its equipment and the many sisters who were qualified teachers, could now take in mentally-handicapped, but she had been rejected without discussion.

Fortunately Lucy, looking quite pretty in her pink nylon dress with her fair hair newly-washed and shining, was comparatively docile during the interview, and Mother Anne agreed to have her for a few afternoons as a trial. If Lucy could fit into the

nursery class she would take her all day—every school-day!
I went home elated.

Martin, when I told him, was not so impressed. More
realistic than I, he said that, though it was reasonable to try, he
did not suppose that Lucy would fit in—however tough their
little boys, he did not suppose they could stand up to Lucy. She
was so strong and destructive he didn't think that their play-
equipment would last five minutes. He even seemed to be
worried lest Lucy should severely injure someone in the first
hour, before the nuns realized her potential. But though she did
seem positively destructive and apparently spiteful at home, I
thought that it might well be because she had nothing to interest
and occupy her, and that with positively-encouraged activities at
nursery school, her energies would be channelled.

Joyously I drove her down, with spare nappies and pants in
her bag, and she happily took my hand to be led in.

The school had plenty of open space, large light class-rooms,
and plenty of equipment. There were slides and climbing frames
in the hall and the garden, sand and water-trays in one class-
room, percussion instruments in another, construction toys in a
third, and lots of nuns to supervise.

Although Lucy was six-and-a-half then she was so tiny, not
having grown at all for the past two years, and her features so
babyish, that anyone would assume her to be about three.
Certainly, when I saw the other nursery children they looked a
sturdy lot beside her, well able to defend themselves.

Mother Anne took us in to Sister Theresa and a small group
of children playing round the sand. Lucy dived into the sand with
the rest and I left her. She took no notice of my going, having
transferred her attention to the sand and the others around it. I
hoped that, at least temporarily, our troubles were over.

When I fetched her all seemed well, though I was surprised to
find her in a different room from the others, with a different nun
to look after her.

Lucy continued to go happily. She obviously enjoyed herself
and was much more quiet and docile when she came home. After
a few days a nun would be there to meet her at the gate, and

when I fetched her she was with a different nun away from the others.

On Friday I went to see Mother Anne as arranged. She told me reluctantly that Lucy could not fit in with the nursery children at all—she was much too rough and boisterous.

She could see, she said, how difficult it must be to manage Lucy in the home, and obviously Lucy was in need of proper full-time training. She urged me to press the authorities to do something about her, and persuaded me to contact again the Society for the Mentally-Handicapped and the Society for Mental Health. And in the meantime, she said, since there was an urgent need for me to get a little relief from her, she would have Lucy for two afternoons a week—not with the nursery class, but separately with a nun to look after her, or rather, a rota of nuns, talking a half-hour period each. Lucy, apparently, needed so much concentrated attention that Mother Anne thought half-an-hour was about as long as one could be sure of staying in command.

Although it was a fee-paying nursery Mother Anne would accept no payment, and she promised to try to continue having Lucy until I had made some more satisfactory arrangement for her.

I fetched Lucy and drove her home. I felt quite numbed. Martin had been right—Lucy could not mix with normal children. What now? It looked as if once again we had got to start writing and phoning and seeking out information and pressing in this corner and that to try to find somewhere for her. But we had tried so thoroughly in the past and it had come to nothing. What more could we do now?

I was too dejected to rush, as I had in the past, to my pen to write to every possible source of assistance. And Martin seemed as despondent as I.

Our days were too long, too harassed. They began when Lucy woke at five and one of us rushed on the instant to get to her before she went on the rampage and disturbed Julia. I changed her nappy and put her sheets in soak and we took her into bed with us for awhile. And from the moment we were up until Lucy was in bed; there was not a single moment in which to relax. When Martin was at work all my time and energy went into amusing and constraining Lucy—and as soon as he was home, he went on duty with Lucy while I washed her nappies and sheets, cooked her special foods, and did the strictly essential household chores. And we anticipated a life-time like that.

It was imperative to get some training for Lucy, whether that was at home or away. If we could get no help from the local authority or the hospital board then we must find a private home, and if necessary mortgage the house to do it. So we summoned our spiritual energy and renewed our efforts.

We wrote simultaneously to the local authority, the hospital board, our MP, the Society for the Mentally-Handicapped, the Society for Mental Health, several major societies with suitable homes, and many private homes. I made several trips to London to see representatives and I visited the day training centre to speak to the head.

It was no use. The local authority would have nothing to do with us, the societies were already overwhelmed, and the private homes were as full as the National Health ones—and who would take a child on an awkward diet, with no bowel or bladder control, when they had a waiting-list of less complicated cases?

Our MP was the only hope. He was sympathetic and said he would make enquiries. Unable to find a solution anywhere else, I pinned all my hope on him.

Daily I watched the clock and waited for the postman, and rushed trembling to examine the letters for the House of Commons postmark. Days and days and days went by—no doubt he had many other claims on his time. Perhaps he was waiting for replies from departments as I had so often waited in the past, but I was not far from despair and I had to hold on to the straw he offered.

So for a time Lucy went down to the convent on two afternoons a week. It was only a small proportion of the total week—but the quietening effect it had on her spilled over to her home activities and she became more amenable. Always when I fetched her I found her happily occupied, even 'working' at something. Sometimes she was in Wellingtons with a rubber apron down to her feet splashing the water, and the sister just laughing and mopping up, or she was hand-in-hand with two sisters walking up and down the steps—they were trying to teach her to go upstairs with two feet instead of one; or she was playing the piano—carefully trying to hit the keys with the same rhythm as the teacher.

They certainly worked very hard at her training, and it was soon evident that they had succeeded in wresting the initiative from her. At home, Lucy took command and we rushed behind taking things away or ducking as she threw them.

But the improvement was not enough for her to join the ordinary nursery class, and there were still too many hours for us to cope.

It was fortunate that Martin was so capable and so domesticated. Often he would bath Lucy or feed her, often play with her or take her out, and when I became too exhausted and distracted to housekeep properly, he would shop on his way home, and cook our supper whenever he was home in the evening.

Often too, he would take and fetch Julia from school—but with the increasing demands on him he had less and less time and energy for talking to her, doing things with her, taking an interest in her. There even came a time when I realized that he was becoming impatient and critical with her—he who had always been so gentle and understanding. What was this situation doing to him? Julia was silent and solemn still—it was evident that she needed more of our time and attention than we were able to give.

And so I continued to look for the postman. And as each day passed without a letter I became more despondent. We had made such a frenzied and prolonged effort the year before to get her some treatment when she was ailing and now that she was healthy again the problems seemed as intractable as ever. Ironically I had brought this situation about myself when I agitated to get medical treatment for her. If I had taken the tranquillizers everyone advised I might have been able to stand aside and watch, I thought bitterly, as, with her mal-absorption undiagnosed, she died slowly of starvation. I would have welcomed her death, but I had not been able to see her suffer.

And now things were different but no better. I was utterly worn out, Martin morose, Julia withdrawn and unhappy. It did not seem that life held much for us. It might be better I thought, if it ended for all of us.

Chapter 16

Our MP was a man new to the district. Young, energetic, enthusiastic, he was already winning for himself a local reputation of being a good constituency man. He held a regular monthly 'clinic' at the Town Hall, where any constituent could go to see him with problems or grievances.

At his next session I went along to see him, taking Lucy with me. I reminded him of my previous letter and outlined the problem again, my voice cracking a bit in my efforts to maintain control.

He listened intently, his secretary making notes, and he promised to do what he could. He had already approached the Ministry of Health, he said, and was awaiting a reply. He was doing everything that he could and would write as soon as he had news. But the comfortable-sounding platitudes met little response from my sceptical mind. I was impatient for action and not at my most reasonable.

I left feeling that I had made a very bad impression. I had complained to him as if he personally were responsible for the situation, and I had made little attempt to thank him for what he said he was already doing. What a fool I felt for having been at all. I felt degraded by having had to go to him to plead for help.

I was rather astonished therefore, when in only a short time I heard both from him and from the Invalid Children's Aid Association, one of those numerous societies I had approached earlier. The association had said then that they would continue to make enquiries and would let me know if anything cropped up, but I had heard that sort of vague hopeful promise so many times before that I paid no heed to it. My MP had also been in touch with them, and they had found a small private home in Wales which would take Lucy temporarily, for a period not exceeding six months, in the hope that a permanent place could be found for her within that time.

That very evening our MP phoned to urge us to accept the place. The fees were high, but he would, he said, do his best to get the fees reimbursed by the authorities, and he hoped that a National Health place might be found for Lucy before her time in Wales was up.

We did accept, though very anxious about the distance from home, the fees, and the uncertainty about the future.

We drove her down, Lucy happy and quiet on the long journey. It was a large ordinary detached house in a quiet residential suburb. We entered with some trepidation, not knowing what to expect, and anxious at having committed Lucy to the unknown. Inside we were reassured by the bright rooms and the noisy babble of children coming from every corner.

Miss Harris, the owner and matron, showed us around and told us that her home was only intended for children under five, but the ICAA had persuaded her to take Lucy because of the impossibility of finding her a place elsewhere. She had, in fact, a few other children over the age-limit, who were all there for that same reason.

There were many cheerful young assistants and trainee nurses who seemed to be occupied amusing and playing with the children as well as tending them.

Lucy was quite at ease and tucked in heartily to the meal they had kept for her. She kissed us, and Miss Harris too, then ran into the garden, eager to join the other children there.

Miss Harris inspired us with confidence. She was one of a handful of people we have met working with the handicapped, who is completely devoted to her work and to the children under her care. Her life was spent with and for them, and she was motivated by their needs. She made one feel very humble.

The next days and weeks were a void. I hardly knew what to do with myself now that I did not have Lucy to dictate my actions. We were still uncertain about how the fees were to be met. As things stood at the moment they were solely our responsibility, so I had to get a job as soon as possible.

The education officer I had met earlier had phoned again in August to ask if there was any possibility of my taking the post as peripatetic teacher of the deaf, but of course at that time it was quite impossible, and so they made other arrangements. Now it was mid-October, well on into a new term. I should be lucky to find a post at all. Yet I did, in a small private school in the next town, and I started immediately.

We continued to communicate with our MP and in late November we heard that Lucy was to be offered a place in Plumfield, the small home we had enquired about before Lucy had been transferred to Haughton.

We were invited to visit and we went together on a misty morning, agitated again by the conflicting emotions of hope and fear—hope that it would prove a fitting home for her, and fear that it might not.

We were ushered in to see the assistant chief nursing officer. He spoke to us for a long time explaining the organization of the home and the daily routine of the children. He boasted to us of how happy everyone was there—staff and children and the older mentally-handicapped women patients who helped on the children's wards. He apologized for the peeling paint and the over-crowded wards and assured us that the patients did not lack for care and attention. He begged us not to condemn the place on the evidence of its material state—especially as, with a recent grant for repairs and alterations, the situation would be greatly improved over the next year or two.

He spoke as if it were all his personal responsibility and concern. A middle-aged man with children of his own, he was yet very involved with the individual care of each of his patients. He was another to add to my collection of anonymous saints.

When we went round the wards we could see the wisdom of his warning. They were quite as bad as he had indicated. My heart sank again. Apart from size it all looked so much like Haughton. Could we condemn our little Lucy to this?

But the staff seemed friendly enough, and there were a number of women patients shuffling about, who smiled and spoke and stared at us curiously. Sister explained that they had come on the

ward to prepare for tea-time: when the children came out of
school, the women would help them with their coats and shoes
and would serve them with tea. They looked happy and eager
enough, although seeing a number of older mentally-handicapped together is always something of an emotional shock.

After all those dreary beds and corridors we crossed the
beautiful gardens to visit the school. The borders were still
colourful with the last chrysanthemums and michaelmas daises
—obviously a few keen gardeners had been at work here. There
were slides and swings and scrambling nets, and a few cages for
pets.

The school-rooms were bright and bustling, the children
noisy and boisterous. The headmistress, gracious and smartly-
dressed, introduced us to her two young assistant teachers,
dynamic, vivacious, and bubbling with enthusiam for their work
and pride in their achievement.

The walls were covered with large collages—the sort of
thing which gives a beautiful effect by having lots of children
stick pieces within large outlines drawn by one artistic teacher.
All the children were busy at different activities, and while we
were there they all left their work to gather round the piano and
sing. This was how they ended every day. It was a strange sound
that they made—but they all sang out heartily, obviously
enjoying it, and those who, like Lucy, could not talk, still used
their singing voices.

We watched as they put their things away, collected their
coats, and were fetched in small groups by the women patients
—their 'aunties'. The children ran eagerly to their own auntie,
some showing a painting or a scruffy piece of folded paper. It
was a delightful scene—the children moving off happily in
different directions jumping and shouting and holding hands
with their aunties.

We stayed some time after the children had gone, talking to
the headmistress, and I thought I had found yet another candi-
date for my collection.

When at last we left the school we went by another path, and
passed the large uncurtained windows of the day-room on the

ward for young teenage boys. We could see them clearly, sitting or standing around idle and pathetic, shoulders slumped and clothes dishevelled, waiting for tea. They must have been too old to have aunties. The male attendant sagged like them, and like them looked bored and blank. Once again I experienced the sickening lurch of the stomach as I was reminded of Haughton.

The conflicting evidence we had gathered was not going to make a decision easy.

We changed our minds a thousand times in the next few days. How could we come to a decision? On the one hand there was the positive advantage of a keen and enlightened nursing officer and a stimulating school, but on the other was those dingy corridors, the lines of iron beds, and the general air of apathy we had seen among the boys as soon as their organized activities were over.

On the credit side again was the fact that they had plans to renovate the place—and too, the warm relationship between the small children and their aunties. But on the debit side the lack of furniture or equipment—the barrenness of even their day-rooms, where presumably they spent most of their weekends—and then the careless dress and general unsightliness of some of the patients.

And what alternative was there?

We did accept, and Lucy went just a week or two before her seventh birthday and Christmas.

Chapter 17

LUCY WAS HOME again for Christmas as usual, and anxiously we studied her for any sign that she was not happy and well-cared-for and kindly treated. But there was none. She was as bright and joyous as when she had been at home. She played as boisterously, she behaved as mischievously; and when the time came to take her back, she returned happily. Surely, we told ourselves, all is well with her at Plumfield.

Nevertheless we subjected Plumfield, its staff and Lucy to close scrutiny over the next few months, but at last we allowed ourselves to believe the evidence that she was in a friendly environment which supplied all her needs—where she could flourish as the green bay-tree.

And flourish she did. She is still there. She is still happy, and has remained so throughout these past four years.

That, I suppose, is really the end of Lucy's story. It was—at least to date—the last of the major upheavals in her life. Little has happened to disturb the placid routine of her days, though a great deal has happened to us.

We are grateful to our MP for his part in obtaining her place at Plumfield. Without his intervention I am sure we should never have had it, nor the cheque to cover her fees at the private home in Wales, which came a few months later.

In fact, after she had been at Plumfield only four or five months we had an ominous letter saying that the superintendent wished to see us, and fear struck us again.

He told us that there had been an enquiry at Haughton shortly after Lucy had left to go to Great Ormond Street and as a result, Haughton was to reduce its numbers. Plumfield had been instructed to 'weed out' any patients who had homes to go to, to make room for some of the overflow.

He asked us how many bedrooms we had, and that seemed to be the only relevant criterion. Many of his patients, he said, came from unsatisfactory homes, often from families who could no longer be traced. A child whose family was known and who could have a bedroom to herself was indeed privileged.

For one bizarre moment I thought that we should have to move away and stop visiting Lucy, or at least move to a two-bedroomed house, in order to retain her place.

But the superintendent was acting on instructions and facing his own dilemma. He was sympathetic when we pointed out the difficulties—in particular the complete lack of training or occupation for her if she came home. He said that he would keep her if he possibly could, but would have to review the situation in six months. Before that time was up Martin himself was dying and we heard no more of it.

Martin's death was so sudden and unexpected—and yet in the deeper recesses of my mind I had feared it for a long time. I had watched the gradual change in his personality as, with each passing month, life became a greater struggle; and when at last his illness was acknowledged it was only weeks before his passing. It was a hurt I cannot speak of here.

Lucy never noticed his going. She was home for the Christmas of her eighth birthday—Martin's last. He played with her persistently—she would not let him do otherwise—but when she came again only a few weeks later and he was gone, she did not notice. She did not feel his death as Julia felt it. Mercifully her limited awareness, her brief memory, spared her that, but Julia will bear the scars of it all her life.

Julia went a year early to the local girls' grammar school—a formal academic situation which some modern educationalists might condemn, but which suited Julia very well. She had been there only a few weeks before Martin went into hospital, and only a term before he died. Nevertheless she coped very well with the immediate situation, and gained a remarkable degree of independence, at least in travelling about and fending for herself, though in personal relationships she was fearful and apprehensive.

There have been a number of changes at Plumfield since Lucy went. The wards have been altered and painted and refurnished —each child has a small open-ended cubicle with a new divan bed and a drawer-shelf-wardrobe unit. The day-rooms have been painted and the reception hall carpeted.

The pets' corner has increased. Now there is an aviary, and rabbits and guinea-pigs, and three donkeys presented by the local Rotary Club.

Lucy was the first to ride on the new donkeys, and seems a natural in the saddle. She is so relaxed she just slumps down in the saddle and lets her mount lead the way.

Lucy has calmed down a little over the years, though she still has a keen sense of fun, and is always in mischief. She loves all the world and expects all the world to love her. She is always ready to kiss, climb up on, be carried or piggy-backed or chased or tickled—by her aunties, by me, or by you. Though if there is a man around she will show a distinct preference for him. A man can lift higher, carry further, tussle more vigorously than a woman—Lucy has learned that for herself.

She is a great favourite at Plumfield. As her nursing officer says affectionately—she livens everyone up and keeps the staff on their toes. And then he goes on to grumble fondly—'Lucy won't walk anywhere these days, she can always find someone to pick her up or give her a piggy. That child never walks the length of the corridor. The staff spoil her, the aunties pet her, and we all do what she wants us to.'

When the responsibility for educating the mentally-handicapped was transferred to the Department of Education in 1971, Plumfield received a grant to expand and re-equip the school. It was also decided that a few of the children, including Lucy, should be sent by mini-bus to a new and well-equipped day training centre about ten miles away. I was delighted about this. Lucy loves car rides so much that a long trip twice a day would be a special pleasure to her—quite apart from the widening of experience which would come from the two environments. Both the school within Plumfield, and the new centre which Lucy attends are run by a dedicated and enthusiastic staff who never cease striving to interest, stimulate, train and enlarge the children under their care.

Lucy's diet has been slowly modified and her bowels have begun to function more normally. I had a few anxious moments after Lucy started her new training centre, when she was sent back to Plumfield on several occasions because of her 'accidents', and it was considered that she might have to return to the Plumfield school—but now she is almost back on a normal diet, and she has gained a good degree of both bowel and bladder control.

Her speech is improving too. Strictly, she has only two words in her vocabulary, 'No' which she uses often and to good effect, and 'Bye-bye' always accompanied by a blown kiss,—but besides this she has a little repertoire of vowel sounds like 'u–o' for come-on, when she is in a hurry, as she almost always is.

When I go to fetch her home she always runs up and hugs me affectionately, waving energetic goodbyes in every direction—and when I take her back she greets the nurses just as eagerly, and as determinedly waves goodbye to me.

At home she is still mischievous and lively and constantly on the go—though more recently she has begun to spend some time drawing doodles with crayons, working at it with great concentration, and studiously coming to show us the result. She makes it plain that we are expected to give it a tick. And then she will go to Julia's old nursery toys, blocks and jig-saws and fitting-shapes, and will work away at them for awhile. Then too she will sing 'la-la', dancing and holding up her arms and demanding that we all join in, holding hands in a circle. Obviously she likes to continue at home the singing and moving rhymes she does at school. And we know when she has seen the dentist, because she examines our teeth.

Still she wants to be off and out—and when she gets bored indoors, will go to the hall pegs and get her coat and struggle into it, and then try to pull us out to do the same thing. And if we resist her she will fetch our coats herself and try to put us into them. With this sort of treatment most people give in after a while.

I remember one occasion, not long before Martin died, when she did this persistently to him, until at last he gave in and went out to the court-yard with her, but he intended to take her walking, and she intended to go in the car. It was an amusing scene—the two of them scuttering back and forth across the courtyard, each trying to impose his own will, Martin trying to be firmly persuasive, pulling Lucy by the hand, and Lucy stamping her feet and shouting, letting forth a stream of unintelligible speech-sounds which could only be interpreted as swearing.

Martin won at last, if you can call it that, when he picked her up in his arms and carried her, but he had to go on carrying her all the way there because she would only walk back. And when she did get back to the courtyard she ran ahead and wrenched at the car door-handle until she got in—and Martin gave up the struggle and drove her twice round the block.

Lucy has her own aunty at Plumfield, Aunty Emma, who is very fond of her. When I fetched Lucy home last Christmas, Aunty Emma was disappointed at having to spend a few days without her. 'I do not know what I shall do without Lucy,' she said, 'I shall miss getting her up in the mornings, and giving her a piggy.'

I have seen another home more modern than Plumfield, and much better equipped, with medical and therapy blocks of every kind, and a much larger medical staff, but not all the equipment and therapy you could devise would make up for Aunty Emma, or for the affection that the small staff at Plumfield bestow upon the children.

Lucy is happy now, and should remain so while she is in a sympathetic environment, though my experience in the past has taught me how uncertain that can be.

Does her present happiness justify her living? It must be weighed against the cost. The cost to Lucy herself in terms of past and possible future suffering, to Martin, to me, to Julia, and to society. The fears I had about the deleterious effect of such a child on parents and siblings were reasonable fears—and they have been realized. Show me a handicapped child, and I'll show you a handicapped family.

My reaction at the time of Lucy's birth cannot be dismissed simply as the effect of post-natal trauma. I had formulated my views about handicapped babies many years before. They were based on a life-time's loving observation of a handicapped sister, and a wide experience of teaching handicapped children. As the mother of such a child and of her sister, I have no reason to change my view.

The sentimental Victorian picture of a mother devoting her life exclusively to her crippled child is an appealing one, easily assimilated and recognizably one we are meant to applaud. But though the mother's action may be commendable as an exercise of Christian virtue, if it does not enable her son to live his life independent of her, to be lovable to others, to be accepted in society, then it is nothing. The most crippled bodies yet have an independent spirit, a need to be loved, and to identify with the community. And if her sacrifice is not too great for her to bear, it may well be for him, for his sister, for his father.

In Devon years ago, walking in the sandstone woodland, I heard an anguished cry—that same quality of sound that sends any mother rushing to protect her child, and later sent me to rescue Lucy from the cold—and when I searched the bracken I found a young rabbit caught in a gin-trap. The fur was torn back from shoulder and leg exposing bone and flesh, and it was panting in the hot sun, crying for relief. There was only one action to take—one which any responsible and humane person finding himself in that situation is obliged to take—and I knew it. I picked up a large lump of that beautiful red rock and held it suspended over its head, while the rabbit continued to cry. Compassion told me clearly what I had to do—but I could not do it.

That I failed to end the life of both the rabbit and Lucy is a measure of my weakness, not my virtue.